DAGGERS
OF THE MIND

DAGGERS
OF THE MIND

Psychiatry and the Myth of Mental Disease

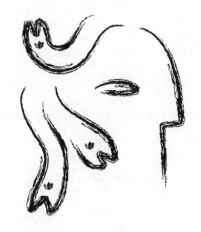

GORDON WARME, MD

ANANSI

Published in 2006 by
House of Anansi Press Inc.
110 Spadina Avenue, Suite 801
Toronto, ON, M5V 2K4
Tel. 416-363-4343
Fax 416-363-1017
www.anansi.ca

Distributed in Canada by
HarperCollins Canada Ltd.
1995 Markham Road
Scarborough, ON, M1B 5M8
Toll free tel. 1-800-387-0117

Page 304 constitutes a continuation of this copyright page.

House of Anansi Press is committed to protecting our natural environment. As part of our efforts, this book is printed on Rolland Enviro paper: it contains 100% post-consumer recycled fibres, is acid-free, and is processed chlorine-free.

10 09 08 07 06   1 2 3 4 5

LIBRARY AND ARCHIVES CANADA CATALOGUING IN PUBLICATION DATA

Warme, Gordon
Daggers of the mind : psychiatry and the myth of mental disease / Gordon Warme.

Includes bibliographical references and index.
ISBN 0-88784-197-X

1. Mental illness. 2. Psychotherapy. 3. Physician and patient. 4. Antidepressants.
5. Placebo (Medicine) I. Title.

RC483.W37 2006   616.89'18   C2005-907428-0

Jacket design and illustration: Paul Hodgson
Author photograph: Joy von Tiedemann Photography Inc.
Text design and typesetting: Sari Naworynski

 Canada Council
for the Arts
Conseil des Arts
du Canada

 ONTARIO ARTS COUNCIL
CONSEIL DES ARTS DE L'ONTARIO

We acknowledge for their financial support of our publishing program
the Canada Council for the Arts, the Ontario Arts Council, and the Government of Canada
through the Book Publishing Industry Development Program (BPIDP).

Printed and bound in Canada

✦ ✦ ✦

Is this a dagger which I see before me,
The handle toward my hand? Come, let me clutch thee —
I have thee not, and yet I see thee still.
Art thou not, fatal vision, sensible
To feeling as to sight? or art thou but
A dagger of the mind, a false creation,
Proceeding from the heat-oppressed brain?

Macbeth

CONTENTS

Introduction 1

PART ONE: MEDICAL RITUALS

CHAPTER ONE: The Love Affair with Science 11

CHAPTER TWO: An Epidemic of Superstition 21

CHAPTER THREE: Drugs Versus Placebos 54

CHAPTER FOUR: The Fallacy of Specific Causes 76

PART TWO: THE VITAL PLEASURES

CHAPTER FIVE: Defeating Guilt 109

CHAPTER SIX: Cleansing and Purging 122

CHAPTER SEVEN: Feasting and Fasting 134

CHAPTER EIGHT: Affirming Who We Are 154

CHAPTER NINE: Decency, Virtue, Righteousness 171

CHAPTER TEN: Firm Conviction 187

CHAPTER ELEVEN: Beauty, Taste, the Arts 202

CHAPTER TWELVE: Reshaping the Soul 212

PART THREE: PSYCHIATRIC CURES

CHAPTER THIRTEEN: Everything Works 239

CHAPTER FOURTEEN: Changing the Theories We Live By 246

CHAPTER FIFTEEN: Placebo: The Secret Healer 259

CHAPTER SIXTEEN: Radiant Oddness 270

Acknowledgements 289

Endnotes 291

Index 295

INTRODUCTION

PSYCHIATRISTS HAVE GOT THEMSELVES mixed up. Hoping for legitimacy, they've bewitched themselves with science, and by neglecting human purposes, they have lost their way. There's particular cause for worry, because many psychiatrists don't know things have gone awry. If we believe what we're told by these science-obsessed psychiatrists, we'll miss out on the most important thing about science: it yields worthwhile results only if there are objective things to study.

Since the late nineteenth century, psychiatrists have studied, researched, and speculated about the biological roots of mental disorders. In recent years, noting its increasing popularity, they've also dabbled in public relations. Aiming to convince people they've zeroed in on the biology of schizophrenia, depression, criminality, and mania, biologically oriented psychiatrists have launched a massive publicity campaign. They believe what they are saying, of course, converted from common sense by a wish for quick cures, by the influence of drug companies, and by the hope for discoveries, the stuff of academic promotion.

To put it bluntly, however, their claims are gross errors, occasionally brazen lies. There's not a scrap of evidence that there are biological abnormalities in any of the so-called psychiatric diseases. Writing in *Neuroscience and Biobehavioral Reviews* about schizophrenia, Albert Wong and Hubert Van Tol[1] have given us the most thorough review article I know, a compendium of the causal theories of schizophrenia that psychiatrists have developed. As they admit, not one of the many dozens of suspected causes of schizophrenia has ever been confirmed.

In an editorial in the *American Journal of Psychiatry,* Dr. Jeffrey A. Lieberman begins with a flat assertion: "It has long been known that schizophrenia is a brain disease." The rashness of this statement is breathtaking. Lieberman, despite what he himself believes, is announcing not a fact, but a manifesto, repeated over the last hundred years by doctors convinced that science and biology are their only destiny and that it is their professional duty to pursue them. Misguided, they've forgotten that "doctoring," playing out a crucial social role, has always been our first obligation.

Dr. Lieberman learned the "schizophrenia is a brain disease" mantra from predecessors who go back to ancient Greece. These proto-biologists lived in unhappy coexistence with their enemies, those who, also since ancient times, have held demons, spirit, mind, or the unconscious responsible for madness.

A few lines after making his flat assertion, Dr. Lieberman acknowledges that modern investigative techniques have come up with nothing: "Although this [investigative] strategy has produced some viable and compelling theories, the pathophysiology of the disease has resisted elucidation by these investigations, in the same way that it has resisted previous efforts to define its histopathology." How, then, can he say, twenty-two lines earlier, that schizophrenia is known to be a brain disease? Lieberman's non sequitur is a stark example of how social practice, more than evidence, influences how we think.

Until psychiatry began publicly promoting its cures — in effect, advertising — this sort of misinformation didn't matter. Previously, having a broad view of the nature of our work, we psychiatrists studied and worried about all aspects of human life: madness, folly, art, deviation, normality. That was how we were trained — or at least how *I* was trained. That generosity of spirit made us uncertain that normality could be pinned down. The upshot was that, alongside oddness and weirdness, conventionality and culture were also deeply studied. This broad view made us close colleagues of philosophers, anthropologists, writers, and English professors.

Now, having joined the world of public relations, psychiatry focuses on popularity. Instead of studying linguistics, philosophy of mind, W. H. Auden, and Wittgenstein, psychiatrists develop programs aimed to popularize their image, projects that appear prominently in hospital brochures — including those of the hospital where I work. Strangely, these projects have little to do with the message of biological causes of mental disease. What has "Strategic Training in Tobacco Use" got to do with serious thought about human life? The important subjects of will and curiosity are forgotten in favour of media-friendly froth like "Ready-to-use Lesson Plans for Drug Education." Although biological words like "gene," "neurotransmitter," and "cerebrum" sound more impressive than behavioural slogans, they are equally irrelevant to serious psychiatric work.

The doctors who work directly with patients are in the right place, but many private practitioners have been converted, crippled by ideas about the imaginary biological disorders they think they are treating. Bad thinking makes for bad decisions. Good thinking, on the other hand, makes doctors hesitate, think things over, dream up better interventions. What worries me is that it's the university doctors — those supposedly committed to rigorous scientific thought — who claim, without evidence, that they have solid answers.

Most, if not all, of the effects of psychiatry are magical. It's risky to say this, of course, because if innocence — some would say medical superstition — is unmasked, my colleagues will become wary, sensing that their skills are being snatched away. It hurts when skills, painfully learned, must be rethought, can no longer be a source of pride, and are redefined as simply interesting and valuable rituals. Just the same, this is the fitting language for our psychiatric wizardry, our placebo cures, the benign and soothing consequences of our medical gestures. The powers of the psychiatrist spring from the important ceremonies and rituals in which we invite our patients to participate. But these words "ceremony" and "ritual" face stiff competition from what is becoming the benchmark: "medical treatment."

✤ ✤ ✤

The greatest danger is that practitioners, if they have been convinced they've got diseases in their crosshairs, will misuse diagnosis. For many psychiatrists, the most dramatic form of madness, schizophrenia, raises the highest suspicion that a biological or scientific cause must be at play. But this can't be proved.

Nor can depression, bipolar disorder, and the various phobias and obsessions be pinned down as valid diagnostic categories. To nail them down as diseases, those claiming that these unhappy states *are* diseases need to show us objective evidence; because so far they cannot, this hasn't been done. To tell unhappy people, without evidence, that they have a disease is unconscionable. Note that, when I say, "so far they cannot [show objective evidence]," I don't mean to imply that I think they ever could come up with such evidence. Because I don't like to think of people who live their lives in unfamiliar, odd, or unconventional ways as sick, I hope the biologists will never be able to surprise me.

In their desperation to prove they've targeted diseases — which of course have to have a cause — some doctors come up with empty explanations. Depressive symptoms are caused by a disease called depression, they say. Or, depression is caused by a depressive gene. Yet no disease or gene has been demonstrated.

Don't be fooled. Psychiatrists *speculate* about undemonstrated genes, hidden infections, chemicals, odd brain configurations, but if challenged, struggle to answer specifics, pointing only to "suggestive evidence." If pressed, they subside. Diagnostic enthusiasts would be consistent only if they admitted there's also suggestive evidence for demons, astrology, and bad karma. As expected, with non-colleagues these medical enthusiasts pull rank, banking on their prestige to make questioners uncertain. Because I'm an insider, I'm immune; with me, colleagues back off. I feel it's my duty as a scientist and doctor to undo the propaganda with which the public is bombarded.

The "suggestive evidence" ploy isn't new. While Joan of Arc marched with her armies, midwives in the entourage had to examine her every day to be sure she was *virgo intacto,* for there was always the risk that, during the night, she might have copulated with an incubus. The membranous hymen, a structure that is variable in appearance, could easily have been perceived as altered, proof of infamous behaviour and a ticket to the fire. In other words, had the midwives said Joan's hymen had changed, "suggestive evidence" would have been found. To prove the same demonic connection, other suspects, men, had their heads and spines examined. "Suggestive evidence" of horns (little bumps on the head) or of a vestigial tail (a suspicious dimple or blotch at the base of the spine) indicated the person was a devil and similarly ripe for burning.

Doctors who take these vague scientific diagnoses seriously have fallen prey to a logical error, the circular argument, an empty sentence in which the predicate is supposed to explain the subject but is really just the same thing. For example:

+ Temper is caused by aggression/anger/rage.
+ Erotic behaviour is caused by a sex instinct.
+ Creativity is caused by an artistic gene.
+ Good judgement is caused by an intact judgement function.
+ Bad judgement is caused by a deficit in the judgement function.
+ Cancer is caused by cancer.

These statements are clearly meaningless. I wish the logical errors of the psychiatrists who think like this could be corrected by giving them philosophy lessons, but they are so enthralled by vacant theories they can't learn.

If skills naive doctors once thought to be proper medical practice turn out to be nothing more than impressive gestures, a cultural and symbolic language, it's hard enough for them to swallow; if the scientific logic they've counted on is unsound, the anguish will be doubled.

The drugs, the electric shocks, and the glib analytic interpretation all need to be rethought.

⁜ ⁜ ⁜

You'll notice I've put all the blame on the doctors and experts. Patients, those who innocently accept our bogus treatments, are off the hook. This is how it has to be. The first principle of social life is that, most of the time, we count on what we're told. I'd be an ass if I doubted my friend's offer to take me to lunch. We count on the dependability of what we are told by friends, newscasters, strangers, and experts.

We especially count on experts — our culture offers an imposing list of them. We make jokes about lawyers being crooks, but we still count on them when needed. Despite our complaints about modern medicine, most people head for a doctor's office when something goes wrong. If we didn't have faith in experts, we'd be on our own for every decision we make. We can't go to medical school every time we're sick, train as a mechanic when our car breaks down, and earn a law degree when we're in legal trouble.

So, when unnecessary car repairs are performed, bad legal advice is given, and sham treatments are offered, blame the expert. Credulity isn't just expectable; to get by in the world it's necessary.

After practising for a while, doctors get to know that much of their work — perhaps most of it — isn't technical or scientific. Words and manner of speaking, they realize, deliver indispensable symbolic messages. It's worrisome that the new breed of pseudo-scientific psychiatrists is less likely than the psychotherapeutically oriented psychiatrists to see that delivering such messages is their main task. It's also second nature for family doctors to know when symbolic wisdom is in order, and to distinguish when something different, a technical intervention, is called for. Strangely, befuddled by envy of the technical wizardry available to colleagues in family practice, surgery, and neurology, psychiatrists are the least skilled at this distinction, so eager to be "real" doctors that they forget that treating biological abnormalities doesn't define a doctor's identity.

Because there is no evidence psychiatry has any specific treatments, and because a high percentage of psychiatric patients get better with every form of treatment, it's clear that, in psychiatric practice, placebos are the prevalent treatment. Therefore, it's no surprise that the doctors most prolific and convinced in their use of placebos are psychiatrists. They are my target because most don't know their treatments are placebos.

The most important lesson psychology can teach us is that psychiatry can't be practised without studying one's own behaviour. Rather than discovering objective things about their patients, psychiatrists struggle constantly with the complicated reactions they and their patients have to one another. Therefore, when I illustrate things from my practice, my personality and beliefs and habits will show up and, just as often, be teased apart and examined. It may be that the most important day-to-day activity of all psychiatrists is the examination of their own biases and preconceptions. Every reader will notice, for example, that I snort at many of the ways of my colleagues. Shouldn't the reader be suspicious of a doctor who is unbending in his position at one extreme of medical opinion? The answer is obvious: yes.

✢ ✢ ✢

The stories I will tell of patients, colleagues, and students are real, although in most cases names and identifying information have been changed. Often, especially when I've wanted to dramatize the interaction between the patient and doctor, I have fictionalized the dialogue.

Note that, throughout the book, I offer many opinions — personal opinions — and less often offer scientific findings. My reasons should be clear already: at best, psychiatric knowledge is a set of tentative opinions. When opinions become unyielding, they are ideology. There is no scientific knowledge of why people act as they do, nor is there scientific knowledge of why people respond well to treatment. This news will be disquieting to some, especially those who have been helped by psychiatrists. My critique will, I hope, alert my misguided colleagues to how they have deceived themselves, not to speak of alerting the public to the misinformation to which they may have been exposed.

PART ONE

MEDICAL RITUALS

CHAPTER ONE

THE LOVE AFFAIR WITH SCIENCE

IF WE'VE DECIDED TO WEAR THE MANTLE OF science, we'd best follow the rules. Popular statements, or those made in a loud voice or with a sweet smile, aren't admitted as science — and, even if the speaker is a psychiatrist, a Viennese accent doesn't help. What counts is evidence: the needle on the instrument must *always* move when the patient carries the diagnosis of schizophrenia, or a brain abnormality must *always* be displayed, or a certain chemical must always be found. Otherwise science is not at work. Suspicions, hints, or the popular "suggestive evidence" cannot claim the important status of scientific statement, not even if that claim is made repeatedly. Nor does the prestige of the person making the statement count.

If scientific tests are passed, findings can be replicated. The X-ray abnormality, the bump on the head, or the strange substance in the urine will always be found.

The fervour for science has changed everything. Among other things, it's made the untidiness of human life unpopular. Nowadays, only science, objectively effective medical treatments, and good sense are acceptable. In the realm of biological disorders — pneumonia, AIDS, coronary artery disease — science has been spectacularly successful as an explanatory and curative tool. I'm distressed when doctors fail to follow scientific method and claim scientific status when they are offering only calcified opinions. Because an unverified opinion that claims to be scientific is worthless — and gives a bad name to science — in later chapters, I will examine the rules that make a scientific claim legitimate.

I am particularly disturbed by the way psychiatrists have embraced what I consider "bad" science. Although convinced they don't practise it, psychiatrists rely on something that has nothing to do with tidiness or science: enchantment. It's our most potent therapeutic weapon. Our rapport with our patients is embedded in wise talk, optimism, and honesty, the medical acts that do much of our therapeutic job. Psychiatrists preoccupied by science thwart their own instincts, liable to be put off balance when patients recover without pills, shocks, injections. Such psychiatrists — and almost every article published in psychiatric journals confirms that academic psychiatry is science-obsessed — have missed what matters most about human behaviour. And when they make scientific claims, no scientific evidence is produced. Good science is one of medicine's principal tools; it shouldn't be misused.

Antidepressants, for example, arguably the most popular psychiatric treatment in recent history, are barely better than sugar pills. Review articles (later I'll make it clear that I'm skeptical of the studies on which such reviews are based) regularly suggest that 71 percent of the effect of these pills is a placebo response.[1,2] This difference is statistically significant, but small enough that, clinically, it doesn't much matter. The slightly higher effectiveness rate of the real drugs, argue the supporters of their use, is due to the antidepressants' specific, curative effects. But it is well known that improvement may be a general, rather than a specific, effect of antidepressants: they stimulate appetite and help sleep in all people, not just the depressed.[3] If we add to this that, because they experience the side effects, many patients know they are getting the active drug, the helpfulness of these drugs becomes even more doubtful. If something that mimics the side effects of anti-depressants is added to the placebo, atropine for example, which dries the mouth in the same way as many antidepressants, the sugar pills work even better.

I believe antidepressants, sugar pills, wise talk, electroshock treat-ment, and being scolded all have the potential to make depressed people feel better. But this is not a scientific claim, just a subjective intu-ition of mine. I also think that going to movies, working out, falling in love, or attending a concert makes lots of depressed people feel better, but this is also not a scientific claim. No science is necessary to say that falling in love makes us feel better; no science is necessary to say that taking pills (herbs, antidepressants, vitamins) makes people feel better.

We're finally stumped by something else: we have no way of meas-uring whether someone is or is not depressed. We have only the patient's opinion, which, in the world of science, counts for nothing. Astrologists, faith healers, and colonic irrigators all report good cure rates, always based on their clients' opinions. This is why citing studies is futile. The supposedly scientific studies — there are thousands of them — all begin with the assumption that the opinions of their patients count as evidence. It's a bit like asking Albanians and Serbians their opinion about the Bosnia-Herzegovina situation and using their answers as evidence. It would be the same with the opinions of conser-vatives and socialists, deists and atheists, opera lovers and rock fans.

It's not clear how, but good treatment effects depend on the rela-tionship doctors have with their patients. To call this superstition sounds unkind, but, hard to stomach or not, it's vital to recognize that we are all credulous and naive. We cling to what we hold precious, including our precious belief that our doctors will help us.

Perhaps, after all, credulity isn't a mistake, and gestures and rituals are neither trivial nor silly. In short, since they help people to get better, I think all types of doctors ought to rethink their uneasiness about the placebo effect. But we mustn't forget that these cures are psychological.

This means that common practices, even though a result of sug-gestion, can still be used. It's okay to prescribe drugs, give electric shocks, put patients on our couches for four hundred hours, but only if we are aware these are medical ceremonies. That they work because of their symbolic power doesn't make them less medical. When known to be ceremonial, these practices are set in aspic — without the rigidity of an ideology; when thought to be definitive, they are set in concrete.

Some are comforted by astrology and homeopathy, others find them silly beyond belief. Neither attitude matters: popular belief comes and goes. It's experts who do harm, doctors who are carried away by fashion, rather than remaining models of cautious wisdom. Sometimes we find it easy to spot charlatans — although those exploited are often hard to dissuade. But charlatans aren't the main enemy. More important are psychiatrists who, when they do their work, don't notice they are using suggestion and fool themselves into believing they have cures.

In his recent book *Historical Dictionary of Psychiatry*,[4] Edward Shorter documents the debut of the word "psychiatry" in an 1808 article by Johann Christian Reil of Halle, Germany. A medical professor, he defined psychiatry as "the third arm of the art of medicine, next to physic [medication] and surgery." Psychiatrists ought to remind themselves that our non-psychiatric colleagues, although skilled at physic and surgery, are also skilled at tending their patients' souls, and that we, the psychiatrists, ought to be proud we've developed this into a special skill. If half a dermatologist's day is spent tending souls, shouldn't we, who do this all day, be particularly good at the skills it requires: making the world comprehensible; being models of courage and calmness in the face of fear; indicating there is a system in place — largely linguistic — that makes the world safe?

Since biology has yielded nothing, the psychiatrists of whom I am complaining are stimulated to try harder, hoping to find hints that, after all, they are on track. Preoccupied, they think desperately that they *must* find signs of biological abnormality. That preoccupation makes them forget that human dilemmas are what matter, and fail to notice what we psychiatrists actually do: talk to people. To strengthen themselves, such psychiatrists should think less about biology, and take into consideration linguistics, symbolic logic, anthropology, and literature, the unacknowledged basic "sciences" of psychiatry. Their concentration on brain anatomy, physiology, chemistry, and histopathology distracts them from the real human issues they must deal with day to day. Biology is fascinating, but rarely useful in our work.

When thinking about worried, unhappy, and strange people, using the language of illness has advantages: it blocks moralizing judgements and makes us think twice when we're tempted to hastily discharge difficult or unattractive people. But the illness model gets misused: to believe psychological unwellness and biological abnormality are synonyms is plainly bad thinking. Although it doesn't occur to those of my colleagues who are duped by biology, were diseases discovered, we'd be out of work. Once discovered, actual diseases are treated by family practitioners and doctors from other specialties. As an example: although mental symptoms are prominent in neurosyphilis and the metabolic disorder porphyria, clear physiological abnormalities have always been easy to detect. But once the cause of these abnormalities was known, neurologists and internists took over. Nowadays, only diseases with no physiological abnormalities fall under the psychiatric umbrella.

To counter the misuse of the words "illness" and "disease," I use as many synonyms as I can. Instead of "schizophrenia," I prefer "madness," but I will also say "insanity," "derangement," or "nervous breakdown." Instead of "anxiety," I prefer "worry," and freely use "unhappiness" as a synonym for "depression." My aim is to sabotage the idea of disease conjured up by words like "schizophrenia," "mania," and "depression." To say someone "has a bee in his bonnet" doesn't mean there is a yellow, stinging insect in his hat, nor does saying someone is "schizophrenic" mean someone's mind is split, or that he has a disease. It's vitally important for psychiatry not to concretize words that are nothing more than interesting — and valuable — metaphors.

✦ ✦ ✦

Rather than appreciating that people recover when treated with everything under the sun, modern psychiatrists are liable to be gullible. It's obvious that almost everything offers comfort to one person or another — drugs, diets, religions, tattoos, strange fashions, enemas, and, as attested to by the successful recruitment of volunteer armies, even wars. This tendency, unless doctors know what they're doing, must not be exploited. But many psychiatrists are inclined to take flimsy evidence of cures at face value, especially the weakest evidence of all: the word of patients who say, "It helped."

This plethora of effects that can be claimed for so many things makes clear that, when I use the word "placebo" broadly, I am claiming that the placebo effect has a deep influence on everything (note, *everything*) humans do. When I make side trips into philosophy and theoretical psychology, I'm trying to underline the important distinction between medical symptoms and something much broader, the character style of our patients. In large measure, after our patients' initial complaints are aired, psychiatric conversations don't focus on symptoms at all, and in the sense that our patients tell us about their understanding of the world, the conversations are about philosophy. Once patients have legitimized their presence in our offices by talking about symptoms, it's their view of life that gets talked about.

If I could change the minds of the sort of psychiatrists I'm worrying about, overcome their naïveté about their good results, and lead them to understand about the placebo effect, they would explain that they were misled by research studies. In other words, the placebo effect doesn't fool just doctors, it fools research studies. That's why it is easy for psychiatrists to stay blind to the ever-present placebo effect: they cite projects that demonstrate that a, b, or c makes people better. What they don't realize is that the various cures they cite are only the currently popular methods; studies of x, y, and z, if administered by healers believed in by their patients, would yield equally good results. Psychiatrists are blind because they are part of a highly organized system of practice, an ideology that, like all ideologies, thinks it possesses the truth.

What *we* believe — everyone, not just psychiatrists — is referred to as reality and good sense; what *others* believe is superstition and folly. What's important is that opinion — or better, mass enthusiasm —

fools naive children and sophisticated psychiatrists alike. Our patients present themselves as representatives of a currently fashionable system of classification: depression, chronic fatigue syndrome, or multiple personality disorders. The giveaway that these conditions are the expression of trends is that, in different epochs, such disorders wax and wane. Those who suffer from such ailments — and they suffer a great deal — would be better served if we would reconceptualize what's going on.

Because its incidence is stable, schizophrenia is more difficult to understand. The stability of this form of madness stems from its archetypal roots; it has played a deeply impressive role in every culture. It is, therefore, thrown up according to the laws of archetypes: every culture bombards its citizens with information about how to be a hermit, a priest, a madman, or a parent, not to speak of how to be a bitch, a puritan, or an artist. Like someone who becomes a lawyer, the madman is sure of his way of life. Like me, the madman is impervious to critique. No matter how loudly he's told — by psychiatrist, priest, or loved ones — that he has an illness, or that he has crazy thoughts, the words bounce off him. His doctors, the ones who say he has a biological disorder, are as sure of their opinions as is the madman of his opinions. Yet biological evidence doesn't exist.

The fragility of the biology argument is given away by the passions that get stirred up when it is challenged. No one gets excited if I doubt the existence of peptic ulcers, although other doctors will think me odd. I'll also be considered boring. But not if I express doubts about schizophrenia. If its biological status is questioned for a moment, an interest group goes into action. I'll be targeted — and I have been — by a high-powered propaganda machine that moves into high gear fast.

Letters and accusations will fly, along with referrals to web sites, experts, and non-existent evidence. Copies of letters sent by the outraged will be forwarded to my hospital and the University of Toronto, where I teach.

In the film *Me, Myself, and Irene*, Jim Carrey portrayed a schizophrenic man. The National Alliance for the Mentally Ill in the United States was dismayed that the film misled the public by not making it clear that schizophrenia is a "severe, biologically-based brain disor-der." It is a remarkable complaint, especially because it is made in uncompromising terms: schizophrenia *is* a brain disorder. The biolog-ical reductionists have made a deadly — and deadening — error. John Churton Collins, a nineteenth-century British literary critic, writing of the superficiality of his era's criticism, says it well: "The scalpel, which lays bare every nerve and every artery in the mechanisms of the body, reveals nothing further."

Fortunately for those who live their lives schizophrenically, chemistry and biology also fail to reveal anything further: there's nothing beyond what the scalpel has revealed. It bewilders me when it's said these per-sons are biologically damaged and diseased. Since that damage and disease are understood to be in contrast to the rest of us — we are robust and intact — the assumption is that they are biologically inferior. Is this an opportunity for social Darwinism and (as documented by Robert Whitaker in *Mad in America*[5]) a renewed outbreak of eugenics?

The rallying cry is science. Ardent schizophrenophiles, the "believ-ers" who love the idea of schizophrenia as a disease, think they've made the right bet, that they're on the side of the angels — and science. The rest of us, those thought not yet to have awakened to modernity and science, are, if you follow that line of thought, primitives. The ped-dlers of schizophrenia as a biological abnormality are correct in saying there are two factions, the superstitious and the scientists, but they've navigated badly: unwittingly, they are the ones who've gone off course, been steered by the treachery of the placebo effect into the choppy waters of superstition, the whirlpools through which they thought they'd long passed.

I like to tackle the science claims, and pointing my colleagues towards the magic of the placebo effect is the most damaging tactic I've come up with. If patients feel better, fooled by the logical fallacy *post hoc ergo propter hoc* ("after this, therefore because of this"), the mis-taken reliance upon temporal succession to prove a causal relationship between two events, naive empiricists will be convinced. Because empiricism is a strong medical tradition, I will have a hard time chang-ing doctors' minds, no matter how damaging my arguments are.

Statements such as "What we see happen is what counts" are empirical. When scientists make such statements, they don't mean the casual "seeing" of everyday life; they are referring to what they can *objectively* observe and evaluate. Because they are nothing more than comments on life in action, psychiatric observations made in the consulting room do not qualify. They are not objectively factual observations. All of us, psychiatrists included, are easily fooled when we don't clearly distinguish between *ordinary* and *objective* observations.

Samuel Johnson's famous argument against Bishop Berkeley's idealism was empirical. No airy-fairy "reality is our ideas" or "reality is merely ideas in the mind of God" argument counted for Johnson. He argued that reality — what we see in front of our eyes — is *obvious*: "I refute you thus," he said, and kicked a stone, hard.

To argue that something is "obvious" is convincing until we remind ourselves that members of the Flat Earth Society still argue their cause on the grounds that their claims are obvious. More ominously, Hitler also "knew" about something obvious: the existence of a Jewish conspiracy. Kicking a stone refutes skepticism, but never-ending human disagreement refutes empiricism, which is only one among many ways of approaching the world. To believe without question in empiricism — raw feel — is just as silly as to believe in skepticism.

Two things immunize one against naive empirical belief: science and critique. Science means evidence-based practice, but the evidence must be objectively demonstrable. That a patient feels better doesn't qualify as a scientific datum. Neither do verbal reports and answers given in responses to a questionnaire — often called a scale — count as evidence. Critique is either an essay on method or a test that yields objective evidence. Placebo effects are "real" in the sense that they make people feel better, but say nothing about a material disease that exists or has been altered.

But the naive beliefs of psychiatrists don't yield easily to scientific rules: much of the time, psychiatrists' superstitions trump scientific facts. Whether we like it or not, beliefs are clung to because they are preferred, supported by evidence or not. Although I prefer work to sloth, my choice of words shows my bias. Many others would disagree and, using their own words, rank placidity higher than obsession. These are matters of taste, the defining feature of superstition: "This is my preferred way of thinking." Some passionately insist that biological causes are the legitimate explanation of human behaviour; others insist that Oedipus complexes, ego weaknesses, and fragmented selves are better illuminators of human life. But these are only explanatory preferences, not scientific theories. People like me must hold our noses and assert that, as preferences, they fall into the same category as astrological influences and the evil eye.

CHAPTER TWO

AN EPIDEMIC OF SUPERSTITION

ON DECEMBER 9, 1484, IN THE FIRST YEAR
of his pontificate, Pope Innocent VIII issued a Bull, *Summis desider-*
antes affectibus, concerning depravity in certain provinces of Germany:

> ... not without afflicting Us with bitter sorrow, that in some
> parts of Northern Germany, as well as in the provinces,
> townships, territories, districts, and dioceses of Mainz,
> Cologne, Trèves, Salzburg and Bremen, many persons of
> both sexes, unmindful of their own salvation and straying
> from the Catholic Faith, have abandoned conjurations, and
> other accursed charms and crafts, enormities and horrid
> offences ... hinder men from performing the sexual act and
> women from conceiving, whence husbands cannot know
> their wives nor wives receive their husbands. ...

The pope was writing about witches. He had appointed his "dear
sons Henry Kramer and James Sprenger, Professors of Theology, of

the Order of Friars Preachers," as inquisitors, and had instructed them to prepare a manual, the *Malleus Maleficarum* (The Witch's Hammer),[1] which codified how to suppress witchcraft. In its three hundred pages the *Malleus Maleficarum* spelled out how to identify and deal with witches — including advice on torture and the use of fiery stakes. The book is, first, a confirmation of the common belief in witches that was held at the time and, second, a set of legal guidelines for their detection and burning at the stake. Among other things, the pope's "dear sons" sincerely argue that one should lie to accused witches in order to trick them into confessing.

Although it's great fun to read, I'm not sure I agree with Montague Summers, the modern editor and translator of the *Malleus Maleficarum*, who, only fifty-five years ago, proclaimed it to be among the most important, wisest, and weightiest books of the world. Or, as Summers also said, "admirable in spite of its trifling blemishes."

The important point isn't the credulity of a modern idiot like Montague Summers; better to ask whether today, five centuries later, in our own way we are as madly credulous as those who lived in the three hundred years during which the *Malleus* was a judicial inspiration. I worry that, when we think we're wiser, more rational, and without superstition, we're at best naive and at worst deluding ourselves. What if we are just as superstitious, but blind to the superstitions that are precious and important to us?

Although this is my prime argument, it's hard to imagine we're as gullible and vindictive as our European forebears, yet the odd world in which we live suggests otherwise. Whose logic, I might ask, should we heed? Palestinian or Israeli? Chechnyan or Russian? Middle Eastern or Western? Capitalist or socialist? My head or my heart? The doctor or the chiropractor?

The last pairing hints at an answer — at least for our society. Because they are identified with science, doctors are on the side of the angels; although we have many traditions, today science trumps every-thing. It's the twentieth and the twenty-first centuries' ace of spades. When I was at university, many women studied Home Economics, but that's not what was written on the neoclassical building at the corner of

Bloor Street and Queen's Park that housed the department. The words still engraved on the pediment make it clear that this was a temple: *Department of Domestic Science.* Now the building has been rented out to the free enterprise of Club Monaco and has become a temple of fashion.

Mortuary science, Christian Science, Scientology, and political science aren't sciences either. Inspired by the spectacular successes of chemistry and physics, morticians, Christian Scientists, Scientologists, and political philosophers improve their image by linking themselves with the prestigious word "science."

Not all skeptics are scientists, but a scientist must be a skeptic. I, for example, am devoted to a skeptical view of the world, but that's not enough to make me a scientist. Nevertheless, a scientist must doubt the way the world has been viewed before his arrival on the scene, or why bother to come up with a brand new theory? Who are the great scientists? All turn out to be dazzling skeptics. The obvious list includes Ptolemy, Copernicus, Galileo, Newton, Einstein, Bohr, and Hawking, adventurers who introduced us to revolutionary views of the world, views so extreme that many of those who expressed them were seen as moral or religious degenerates.

Rather than doing revolutionary science, most scientists work out the details of what their adventuresome predecessors have come up with, a work called "normal science." Just as skeptical in their aims as their earth-shaking ancestors, those who do normal science are suspicious in principle, busy trying to disprove the theories they are working on. If the evidence they come up with doesn't support the bright idea — the theory — it becomes an error, soon forgotten or relegated to the category of historical peculiarity. Such work is not to be sniffed at; I'm happy the principles of Newtonian physics have survived the severe tests of normal science and that I can safely live in a high-rise building designed according to those principles. These designs were painstakingly worked out by many generations of Isaac Newton's followers.

Like all scientists, doctors discover things by coming up with bright ideas, then confirm or disprove them using the principles of evidence and prediction. They are then worked out in detail by physicians who follow. As in any scientific work, if the details don't confirm what's been proposed, the bright idea becomes an error and is forgotten. Except in psychiatry.

Psychiatry has had two bright ideas, both of which have been around since ancient Greece. The first idea, already clear in the school of Hippocrates, is that madness is caused by bad biology. This theory has not yet yielded to the attempts of psychiatrists to find evidence. Were the madman's biology amiss, my opinion is that the secrets of madness would, long ago, have capitulated to our scientific efforts and yielded up evidence of abnormality in the body, brain, or physiology. Since there's not yet a scrap of such evidence, the biological bright idea is unfounded, and should not, as it now does, occupy centre stage. It should, many years ago, have been recategorized as questionable.

The most popular recent candidate for the title of Biological Cause — abnormalities in the brain's neurotransmitters — is also the most recent disappointment — or so I'm told in the corridors of the Centre for Addiction and Mental Health (CAMH) by colleagues who, like me, are disappointed by unsubstantiated claims. Neurotransmitters are chemicals that are used to relay, amplify, and modulate electrical signals between a neuron and another cell. In schizophrenic patients these chemicals are assumed to act abnormally. But after years of research, no abnormalities in neurotransmitter functioning have ever been demonstrated in psychiatric patients. Despite many claims, I cannot find one substantiating article. Instead I find statements of opinion and belief, especially striking when used by one of the most senior psychiatrists in the United States, editor of the *American Journal of Psychiatry*:[2]

+ "Dopamine was the first neurotransmitter to be discovered [sic] as a contributor to the symptoms of schizophrenia. Several lines of evidence *have suggested* that dopamine is important in this illness."
+ "Clinician scientists *now think* that schizophrenia occurs as a consequence of a much more complex chemical imbalance that includes multiple neurotransmitter systems that interact with and modulate one another."

✦ "What does this pattern of response *suggest* about the neurochem-
istry of depression? . . . *likely . . . is the possibility* that these two
neurotransmitters . . . work together to achieve an overall balance."
(my italics)

It's hard to call up negative evidence, evidence that doesn't exist. It
is therefore a relief that the American Psychiatric Association, after
being pressured and threatened by anti-psychiatry activists, has admitted that there is no biological evidence of biological abnormality in any
psychiatric disorder.[3]

✤ ✤ ✤

The second psychiatric bright idea, perhaps first explicit in Greek
tragedy, is that madness is due to spiritual disquiet. That idea is quite
another matter. There is no reason to believe that the human spirit —
psychology, mind, thinking, hoping, feeling, striving, or whatever
other symptoms you prefer — should yield to objective study. It is, in
principle, not at home in the world of science. That's why I didn't
include Sigmund Freud in the list of great scientists. Although he
thought he was one, he was really *"ein Dichter,"* a word commonly rendered in English as "a poet." But it means much more: "poet,"
"novelist," "he-who-tells-vital-tales."

There's no doubt that belief in witchcraft was one of the great hysterias; more and more I suspect that a badly misunderstood version
of science has been enlisted as another of the great hysterias.
Administrators! Clinical psychiatrists! Research assistants! Please
leave science to the scientists.

✤ ✤ ✤

Four decades ago an attempt was made to improve the blood flow to
the heart of patients suffering with angina pectoris — heart pain — by
making an incision in their chests and tying off the two internal mammary arteries. The results were sensational: 90 percent of patients had

good pain relief. But the researchers also made incisions in the chests of patients *without* tying off the arteries, and the sham operation turned out to be just as effective. The procedure, internal mammary ligation, was abandoned. Reliable studies suggest that migraine headaches, back pain, post-surgical pain, and rheumatoid arthritis all respond well to placebos.

It's common to believe the placebo effect is an imagined disappearance of symptoms, that a belief in the treatment leads to subjective improvement. But placebos often produce physical changes as well: when asthmatic patients are told they are inhaling a bronchodilator, their bronchial tubes expand. Blood pressure, skin temperature, cholesterol levels, heart rates, and contact dermatitis are all affected by placebos.

These effects aren't trivial. In its opposite version, the nocebo, its psycho-physiological effects can be lethal; the fear of death can lead to a person's actual death. More common, and upsetting to its victims, is when fear that he might miss the net leads a hockey player to choke, or fear of fainting leads someone to faint, or fear of forgetting his lines causes an actor to . . . forget his lines. There are many cross-cultural examples. One is voodoo death, in which a person dies when a powerful cultural figure points a bone at him. I remind myself that belief has two effects: positive belief (placebo) heals; negative belief (nocebo) sickens or kills. Both good and bad effects have deep cultural roots. In detail and with great force, all cultures teach citizens how to respond to suggestion.

. ✢ ✢ ✢

Even if doctors know they are applying coloured water, warts disappear, a treatment known to Tom Sawyer, who also understood that the ritual had to be conducted exactly as prescribed:

> "Barley-corn, Barley-corn, injun-meal shorts,
> Spunk-water, spunk-water, swaller these warts." And then
> walk away quick, eleven steps, with your eyes shut, and then
> turn around three times and walk home without speaking
> to anybody. Because if you speak the charm's busted.

Expectation accounts for all theories of how the placebo effect works. The release of endorphins, learning, and conditioning all follow upon the patient's expectation that the doctor or healer has great power. Countless changes — nerve functioning, chemistry, and personal will, both conscious and unconscious — are induced by those wonderful expectations.

This is a far cry from scientific materialism, the reduction of everything human to biology. No scientist should make the reductionism error, but modern psychiatrists blithely embrace a philosophical doctrine that works fine for the mechanics of building bridges, but is useless for the aesthetics of a bridge, for relativity and quantum studies, or for sociology and psychology: people are composed of stories, not atoms.

The psychiatrists currently in the ascendancy in the universities act as though they've never heard of theoretical frameworks other than anatomy and neurophysiology (the tangible medical equivalents of physics and chemistry). It's a commonplace that materialism is only marginally useful for studying human behaviour; I'd be a madman if I thought about chemicals when my grandson tells a good joke. Behaviour is just too maddeningly complicated to be understood in simple terms. The instant the words chemical and neurotransmitter are uttered, the soul disappears; psychobabble has been replaced by biobabble. On the ground — and in the work of good theorists — behaviour is always understood psychologically. Why? Because human behaviour and psychology are the same thing.

✣ ✣ ✣

As I've said, psychiatry has twin roots, the histories of both extending back to ancient Greece. From the time of the earliest historical records, some thought madness (only overt madness and flamboyant hysterias were of interest until the twentieth century) was due to physical causes, often causes in the brain. Others thought madness to be dynamic, a result of personal or alien forces that, rather than being blindly somatic, were intelligent and possessed the madman with some purpose in mind. Henri Ellenberger's *Discovery of the Unconscious*,[4] written in 1970 and still a masterpiece of psychiatric history, traces these two historical threads into the modern era.

Psychiatrists in the nineteenth century broke decisively from demonism and exorcism and made tentative moves towards science. Exorcists had tapped into the placebo effect easily and had had terrific results: their patients got better just as modern patients do. But it wasn't until Anton Mesmer in Germany became interested in magnetic diseases, in the late eighteenth century, that physical causes were systematically assumed to be present in cases of hysteria and madness. Mesmer cured thousands of people, cures that displaced the exorcisms previously used to cure the mad. Nowadays we'd consider Mesmer a quack; he cured people of all sorts of ailments, in groups, supposedly by activating a magnetic fluid he thought to be present in all people but blocked in those who were unwell. After being ostracized in Germany, he practised in France, still sure he'd discovered a real, physical cause for hysterical paralysis, an abnormality in something he called "animal magnetism."

Hippolyte Bernheim, who practised in the city of Nancy in France in the nineteenth century, paid serious attention to hypnosis, an outgrowth of Mesmer's magnetism. Over the years, however, Bernheim stopped trying to conceptualize a mysterious substance/fluid/energy to explain his helpful effect on patients: he attributed his good results to suggestion. Bernheim was right, although the innocent word "suggestion" doesn't convey the importance of Bernheim's simple idea. He'd noted that patients get better because of the placebo effect (though he didn't use that word), the suggestive effect of the doctor, the culture's designated healer.

But Berheim's straightforward — and obvious — "suggestion" hypothesis gets less attention than impressive-sounding things like animal magnetism, synaptic clefts, and serotonin. Indeed, Bernheim is now mostly forgotten. Nor, I might add, do modern-day naive observations, deadly accurate though they may be, sound as impressive as do important-sounding words like unconscious, complexes, and libido. I have a hunch that psychiatric symptoms are "suggested" by the culture (which would explain the "trends" in disorders), that a clearer light is thrown upon psychiatric disorders if we keep suggestion in mind. Furthermore — and this I've already made clear — our treatments of these disorders succeeds because of the same phenomenon: suggestion.

Emil Kraepelin and Sigmund Freud, only a few years later, at the end of the nineteenth century and into the early twentieth, were the best-known representatives of the two major schools of psychiatry that eventually evolved: solid material causes on the one hand; intangibles, like suggestion and hope, on the other.

Kraepelin, who worked in Heidelberg and Munich, was the first to make the strong claim that madness was an abnormality of the brain, and he did so backed up by as little evidence as modern psychiatrists bring forward. Even then, such theories were called *Hirnmythologie*, "brain mythology." Kraepelin's errors are easier to understand than are the errors of modern psychiatrists; until the 1930s, half the population of psychiatric hospitals actually had biologically damaged brains: neurosyphilis; what we now call Alzheimer's disease; atherosclerosis of the arteries of the brain.

Not a therapeutic enthusiast, Kraepelin emphasized classification. Prior to Kraepelin, psychiatry had been interested in a large and heterogeneous group of psychiatric disorders — mania, catatonia, melancholia, hebephrenia, paranoia — not thought to be related to one another, but which Kraepelin catalogued into two groups: dementia praecox (the first name for schizophrenia, suggestive of a premature deterioration of mental life) and manic-depressive illness. The classification was based on the course and outcome of these so-called diseases: patients with the former disease, dementia praecox, had an inevitable downward course; those with the latter, manic-depression, recovered spontaneously. Apart from conscientious humanitarian care, treatment wasn't an issue.

In Vienna, Freud laboured under the opposite illusion. Rather than believing in mythical physical causes for madness, he devised an ingenious mythical psychology, a set of conflicting mental forces: "psycho-physics." These, he claimed, caused a *mental* form of pathology. Because he had good treatment results, he shared the conviction of modern psychiatrists that patients have diseases that doctors are supposed to "cure," and that his psychoanalytic treatments did just that, cured them. Kraepelin postulated material diseases; Freud postulated spiritual diseases.

Because the biological psychiatrists have convinced themselves that there are physiological causes for psychiatric disorders, they don't really think further about what might be going on. Because it's been decided *in advance* that the patient is biologically tainted, thinking is superfluous. In other words, a particular philosophical position is held as dogma. Phenomenology — careful observation — has been replaced by a naive form of materialism.

The debate between materialistic and dynamic psychiatry continues, and is likely to go on forever. To a materialist, depression is caused by genes and abnormal chemistry; to a dynamic (analytic) psychiatrist, depression is caused by complexes, bad parents, and thwarting cultures. Because of the human tendency to concretize metaphors, some psychiatrists will always forget that when we say a madman is "sick," we are using a figure of speech; they therefore turn sickness into something real. Waves of enthusiasm will lead psychiatrists to swing back and forth between the two misreadings of this metaphor: abnormal brains versus abnormal minds. The popular enthusiasm, currently overrepresented in academia, is for abnormal brains. Improperly, those who make this error are making moral judgements; because they don't like it that people suffer, are fools, act peculiar, they use a euphemism: disease. Euphemisms are thin lies, bad for the character. Only the faint-of-heart find intolerable something that is a commonplace: human folly.

✦✦✦

Another fashion — both psychiatric and public — is to consider the everyday trials of living to be illnesses. Read a novel, see a film, attend the theatre, and you'll see that most problems are just ordinary human life. The novel, film, and play can be high art or kitsch: all consistently focus on what human life is like.

Jim Windolf, executive editor of the *New York Observer*, in an article published in the *Wall Street Journal*,[5] zeros in on the American sickness epidemic — the perception-of-illness epidemic.

He tells us that, according to various sources, nine and a half million adult Americans suffer from attention deficit disorder, more than ten million have seasonal affective disorder, and five hundred thousand more have chronic fatigue syndrome. Add in fourteen million alcoholics, five million with severe mental illness, two and a half million with multiple chemical sensitivities (they daren't touch Windex, says Windolf with a wink). But these figures, he says, are trumped by the National Academy of Sciences, which claims thirty-seven million Americans have increased allergic reaction to chemicals. Social phobia, fifteen million; depression, fifteen million; borderline personality disorder, ten million; restless leg syndrome, twelve million; obsessive-compulsive disorder, almost five and a half million; manic-depressive illness, two million; sex addiction, eleven million. Total: 77 percent of Americans. Windolf wryly adds that the figure is higher if we include alien abduction, road rage, or Internet addiction. I wonder how Windolf missed drug addiction, gambling, and neurosis?

What in the world is going on? Every measure of social welfare indicates that, in the last fifty years, we've become drastically healthier, and live longer in better houses. Our IQs are climbing, and crime is decreasing. Yet, when they are asked, the graph shows that people who say they are "very happy" are in decline and, as we all know, incidence of depression is soaring. I know that humans are said to be the sick animal, but surely it's against every psychiatric morality to encourage such pessimistic thinking. Somehow, we doctors have stopped encouraging our patients, bucking them up with our confidence and enthusiasm, and are instead making ominous pronouncements about diseases. As well, all too often, I hear colleagues say, "Depression is still underdiagnosed." Do these people promote this madness because they are dolts and louts, caught in a communal hysteria they themselves have inspired, yet ought to stand against?

This hurricane of psychologically spawned illnesses — sometimes called "media disorders" — has generated a parallel hurricane of placebo remedies. Countless drugs, support groups, and therapies give succour to these sufferers. The sort of explanation we seek to give shouldn't demean them (among other things, it's bad medical ethics), and, if we tell people their bodies are tainted with real, material disease, that's what we risk doing. Perhaps we could say they're slaves of fashion, or, more accurately, that they are skilled in the current language of suffering. Perhaps doctors should adapt to this language, not take the symptoms as evidence of actual physical pathology, but of suffering, and reply in kind: respond compassionately with symbolic words and gestures. Although it leads to no objective changes, symbolic talk is a real treatment, and pills, tonics, and injections only distract us from our main task. The most medical thing we can do is to know what we are doing.

I've been struck by a pattern. When they phone our clinic, patients with multiple personality disorder often ask for a doctor who has particular knowledge of that disorder (patients with dissociative disorders, who tell alien-abduction stories, do this, too). They think of themselves as unusual, special, and amazing, demonstrating a sort of pride that is aided and abetted by the media and by a few impressionable doctors. Some of these patients have asked me directly whether I would contact the media, priests, and police officers that they'd run into when in one of their multiple personalities. When, rather than treating them as freaks, I try to talk to them about why they think as they do, these patients often stop. What they're doing, of course, is running from psychiatrist to psychiatrist, hoping to be considered astonishing or a rarity. Since humouring them means they aren't treated as fully human, it's wrong for a doctor to agree.

I worry that the culture of psychotherapy — I'm one of those who promote this fashion — has legitimized the towering self-obsession that lies behind this noisy complaining. The consequence is a culture of complaint in which many people are frightened, and a small subgroup, made up of bellyachers and the litigious, are invited to step forward. This culture also silences skeptics: if we don't agree that they are ill, we're branded as heartless and uncaring. Analogously, in a culture of self-improvement, there's no need to enlist the excuse of illness:

many of us upgrade cosmetically, tamper with our brain-chemistry, our physiology, and our faces, determined to improve on nature.

There's a rampant belief that we ought to have flawless health, live to one hundred without aging, and, in the hands of our psychiatrists, be made conflict-free, and content. This isn't what a good psychiatrist is after; our goal is to help our patients get a bit wiser — wistful intelligence is what I like to call it — and, as often as not, this is a product of the thing people try to get rid of: conflict.

Peace of mind is fun to talk about, good for idle daydreams, but deadly for a living, breathing soul. Seeking freedom from conflict is partner to other worrisome medical enhancements: taking steroids and growth hormones to beef up athletes, and to give them heart disease later on; swallowing fertility drugs that cause the ovaries to gush ova into fallopian tubes; inserting genes to enhance intelligence. Who gets those genes? My children? The children of the poor? Never mind that intelligence is a doubtful category; it's the diabolical thinking that worries me: I don't want my sweetheart to love me because Puck sprinkled fairy dust into her eyes.

The cornucopia of disorders is typical of cultural passions/hysterias; they appear in a multitude of guises, they are said to have a multitude of causes, and a multitude of remedies are available to "cure" them. Four hundred years ago, in his *Anatomy of Melancholy*,[6] Robert Burton listed the causes that bred melancholy:

> beef and pork are suspect, goat's flesh and all venison; hare is hard of digestion, although some say that "hare is a merry meat, and that it will make one fair," as Martial's epigram testifies to Gellia. . . . Most fowl and all fish are discommended, a great number of vegetables . . . much bread, and all black wines, and beer is most unwholesome.

And as for cures:

> Seventeen particular cures, mentioned by Aristotle, "for brevity's sake I must omit": . . . Thus music is a roaring Meg

against melancholy. "Many herbs are wholesome for it . . . all their study should be to make a melancholy man fat, and then the cure is ended . . . two or three holes bored in the head, to let out the noxious vapors . . . calculate spherical triangles, square a circle, cast a nativity," or let him read books of mathematicks, metaphysics, and school divinity.

Anticipating modern hysterical fashion, the list of causes and cures goes on and on. As opposed to modern psychiatrists — who accept a cornucopia of treatments for every psychiatric disorder — Burton knew that his lists of treatments didn't make sense. He was recording his era's practices, not advising. In a brilliant review of *The Anatomy of Melancholy* in *The New York Review of Books* in 2005,[7] Charles Rosen chose to quote the following portion of Burton:

> Who can sufficiently speake of these symptoms, or prescribe rules to comprehend them? . . . If you will describe melancholy, describe a phantasticall conceipt, a corrupt imagination, vaine thoughts and different, which who can doe? The foure and twenty letters [of the alphabet] make no more variety of words in divers languages, than melancholy conceipts produce diversity of symptoms in severall persons. They are irregular, obscure, various, so infinite, *Proteus* himselfe is not so divers, you may as well make the *Moone* a new coat, as a true character of a melancholy man; as soone finde the motion of a bird in the aire, as the heart of a man, a melancholy man.

And:

> And who is not a Foole, who is free from Melancholy? Who is not touched more or lesse in habit or disposition? . . . And who is not sick, or ill-disposed, in whom doth not passion, anger, envie, discontent, fear & sorrow raigne?

✛ ✛ ✛

Let's call a spade a spade: psychiatry's various treatments are superstitions, too. But if the biology-enthralled psychiatrists can convince the public — and themselves — that they are scientists, they can sidestep any awareness that even science is a belief system, and that the accusation of superstition works only if beliefs are uncommon or culturally unexpected. The idea they want to get clear is that science is special, different from other ways of approaching the world. Science does have unique identifying characteristics, valuable in certain circumstances, but not applicable to psychiatry; our profession doesn't deal with objective facts, the precondition of scientific practice.

Unfamiliarity should not be the element that makes superstitions disquieting; concern is reserved for superstitions that do harm. Of those, I have two examples. The first example is superstitions that blame our troubles on others, things like racism and unjust prejudices. The second example is psychiatric. If our treatment is a healing ritual — if we are aiming for a placebo effect, in other words — it should not have the potential to cause dangerous side effects. Powerful drugs are the best example. This danger is invisible if we believe our psychiatric successes are scientific.

✛ ✛ ✛

Hysterical excitements are all superstitions, many of them wonderful. But I worry about people who believe concretely that their hysterical fears are real, as in "I've got a disease called post-traumatic stress disorder." Trauma is real, at times devastating. But this is only one among many stereotypes about how we are to react to trauma. There are other stereotypes just as real and just as honourable: the stiff upper lip (demonstrated by the British, Scandinavians, Northern Germans, and half of North Americans) is the well-bred response of some people, as legitimate and honourable as feeling traumatized. To be expressive and vocal (like Southern Germans, Italians, Arabs, half of North Americans) is the equally well-bred style of others. But since the British reaction doesn't fit the "post-traumatic stress disorder" stereotype, we are at risk of thinking the Brits are weird or unwell (or failing to grieve properly) because they don't react noisily. But surely none of these reactions are diseases.

Indulge preferred rituals, I say. Northerners, bravely stiffen your lips. If you can't, take assertiveness training, attend a military school, begin bodybuilding. Southerners, bravely display your despair. Put the backs of your hands to your foreheads and swoon away — and if you can't, psychiatrists will help, as will smelling salts, tonics, and rest cures.

Because distressed people can be *very* distressed, humour is risky. But there are lots of serious words other than "traumatized" that we can and ought to use: miserable, sick, devastated, crushed. These important metaphors mustn't be misunderstood as being concretely true. If I've experienced an awful event, and say I'm devastated or crushed, this doesn't mean I've been laid waste, nor have I been crushed flat as a pancake. These are evocative metaphors. Nor, if I say I'm sickened by what happened, does it mean I've got a disease. Yet many of my psychiatric colleagues have taken the "sick" metaphor literally and decided that, if I'm a wreck after something awful has happened, I have a disease. This isn't just harmless silliness. To tell me I have a disease makes me helpless, robs me of the internal pep talks I would ordinarily use to get myself going. It also robs me of my pride: I'm not, I'm being told, a person able to cope with life independently, to deal with things.

The definition of superstition that follows is neutral, but our usual habits of thought attribute silliness to it, even though it's one of the most important and defining things about humans:

> Superstition: an irrational but usually deep-seated belief in
> the magical effects of a particular action or ritual, especially
> in the likelihood that good or bad luck will result from per-
> forming it.

We think we've outgrown superstition, convinced we're smart and rational, aware of science, the way of thinking that doesn't buy into the folly of such things. For those who think this way, the fly in the oint-ment is that blind belief in science is also a superstition. Philosophically sophisticated scientists know science has little to do with discovering the truth; science is practical, and finds ways to make sense of the world and to do certain things — nothing more. When scientists test their theories, they aren't testing the truth of their theory. They want to know whether, for now, the theory is a good one, and are always ready to abandon theories that don't pass their tests. In practice, theories that stand up well to testing are pursued because they are practical, even something as mildly "practical" as being able to make accurate predic-tions of the weather. Unfortunately, some scientists misunderstand and, like priests, think the products of their work are true.

If it's time to call a spade a spade, we must acknowledge supersti-tion to be inconsistently visible. Sometimes we see it in ourselves, but superstition is most starkly visible in others. In societies with which we are unfamiliar, cultural rituals seem bizarre, silly, in need of correc-tion. The accusers in the Salem witch trials of 1692 were typical because they noted, not what they themselves did, but what others did. Arthur Miller, in the 1950s, was appalled when friends had their careers damaged by the McCarthy Senate hearings. To his horror, some co-operated with the investigations and confessed, to save themselves and their families. His play *The Crucible* nails down the perfect analogy between the Salem trials and the House Committee on Un-American Activities hearings: the McCarthy witch-hunt was as profoundly ritualistic as its precursor 250 years before. In *Timebends*,[8] his autobiography, Miller points out that:

> The main point of the [McCarthy] hearings, precisely as in seventeenth-century Salem, was that the accused make public confession, damn his confederates as well as his Devil master, and guarantee his sterling new allegiance by breaking disgusting old vows — whereupon he was let loose . . . The Salem prosecution was actually on more solid legal ground since the defendant, if guilty of familiarity with the Unclean One, had broken a law against the practice of

witchcraft, a civil as well as a religious offense; whereas the offender against HUAC could not be accused of any such violation . . .

The mad epidemic of modern illnesses is one of *our* hysterical superstitions, a phenomenon visible to many of us. But most of our own superstitions, unless we exert great mental effort, are invisible. My argument is that medical superstitions are essential, but, if not blessed with a respectable label like science or treatment, are considered to be foreign and are therefore viewed with skepticism. Once a mainstay of medical treatment, bleeding patients is now laughable, an amazing bit of medical humbug; psychoanalysis, patients lying on a couch and free-associating, now raises the eyebrows of young doctors, but, not yet having been fully assigned to historical quaintness, is still widely practised by psychiatrists like me. Psychiatric drugs, however, are only recognized as a fad by occasional skeptics; even psychotherapeutically oriented psychiatrists are tempted to accept the prevailing opinion that these drugs have specific effects, and, by prescribing them, to neglect the interpersonal rituals at which they are expert.

The torrent of placebo cures is testimony to our need for magic, although there's a better way of saying it: our need for soul-stirring cultural ceremonies. Those who take communion, prostrate themselves to Allah, or kiss the Torah as it passes by are participating in precious cultural rituals, as are those who take herbs, have their innards irrigated, or believe depression can be scientifically understood.

What is commonly called hysteria is the most visible example of how behaviour is a product of cultural influence and suggestion. The word "hysteria" is tricky, and is mostly used for behaviours on the fringe of respectability. It's considered good to be masculine or feminine, but excessive bodybuilding and wearing revealing clothing are marginal behaviours liable to earn censure or mockery. When we see extremes of masculine behaviour, we're tempted to say "he's insecure" or "he's compensating"; however, "hysteria" is the preferred word when commenting on extremes of feminine behaviour. The important point is that, for both men and women, when gender-specific behaviours are emphasized beyond a certain threshold, and when we call it hysteria, we are making moral judgements.

"Hysteria" refers to many things, mostly a pattern of actions considered excessive. The perception of artifice mentioned above inclines us to think of hysteria. Although useless as a medical category, doctors still use the word when speaking casually. Psychiatrists use the word two ways. The first use is in reference to a personality type, a way of life: great enjoyment of gender, demonstrated in supremely masculine men and wonderfully feminine women. But there is always of hint of criticism.

The second use of the word "hysteria" is for the passions stirred in groups by important causes like the Beatles or Wagner, and by ideologies that range from liberty to revolution to racism. Of more importance to doctors are media-inflamed group passions that foster a belief in disorders like depressive disease, multiple personality disorder, panic, and widespread and puzzling somatic complaints. These terms refer to real suffering and unhappiness, but, because they are ordinary human states, should not be considered diseases that could be cured or will ever be wiped out.

Professionally, psychiatrists don't talk about hysteria any more: it's been erased from our official language: no such diagnosis exists in the *Diagnostic and Statistical Manual*[9] of the American Psychiatric Association (DSM-IV). But in the corridors of hospitals and at lunch, he or she, the hysteric, is alive and well, most commonly in the person of the highly feminine woman. Of Marilyn Monroe we say, affectionately, "She's not dead, you know." In many of her incarnations the hysteric is a goddess of beauty, such as Helen of Troy, for example, the most beautiful woman who ever lived, not to mention her countless other appearances in her various archetypal roles: Madame Bovary, Salomé, Josephine Baker, Marlene Dietrich.

Male hysterics, usually warriors, are also well loved: Muhammad Ali, the genius of trash-talk, fighting in and out of the ring; Pierre Trudeau, intellectually combative, at the drop of a hat ready to quarrel, perfecting the picture of hysteria by being brushed with effeminacy;

Clint Eastwood, saying, memorably, "Make my day." Also Achilles, Robin Hood, and Spiderman. Who else but a hysteric would wear a costume like Batman and Superman?

When a woman's hysteria is overdone, the signs are well known: swooning, paralyses, squeals, gagging. Totally out of hand she's a bitch, a wanton, a whore, a seductress. Typically, we think that when a man's hysteria has gone awry, it should resemble female hysteria; we don't like to notice that the signs of overdone male hysteria are also common and obvious: bullying, machismo, boasting, dispensing smacks and slaps. Out of hand he's a looter, rapist, and pillager. The mobsters in *The Godfather* and *The Sopranos* are hysterics. The vamping transvestite and the camouflage-clad lesbian, on the other hand, are only parodies.

In short, when we use the word "hysteria" we're usually referring to behaviour that's intimately linked to gender. It's not a medical category. But, because it points to our intolerance of marginal actions, it is an important category, especially important when we consider, first, the widespread over-treatment of minor psychiatric symptoms and, second, the forced hospitalization and treatment of extreme oddness, madness, and unconventionality.

✢ ✢ ✢

Chronic fatigue syndrome has, in recent years, been thought a newly discovered disease. But it was commonly diagnosed more than a hundred years ago, and was then called neurasthenia. The signs and symptoms in the late-eighteenth century were identical to what's now described. Neurasthenia, the doctors decided, was due to depletion of nervous energy in the brain; when I was a student, the same disorder was said to be due to depletion of *psychic* energy in the brain. But no causes have ever, then or now, been discovered. There are no objective findings; we know only that certain people feel tired — very tired.

Because there is no treatment, to tell these patients they have a disease — and that's what happens — is to invite them to give up. Thinking they know why they are fatigued, there's no reason for them to think further, to wonder, struggle, hope there is more to understand. If we had one, a widely accepted placebo would be terrific: take the waters (at Baden Baden, perhaps, or at Radium Hot Springs in British Columbia), herbs, vitamins, mountain air. But doctors now don't believe in these things, so they're not sure what to do.

The best placebo treatment for chronic fatigue syndrome is psychotherapy. First, it's the most popular of our era's placebo treatments, second, doctors believe in it, and third — this is the most important reason — because it fits with our culture's way of thinking: introspection is highly valued and widely encouraged. Even theatrical and literary characters are thought admirable if they spend time in introspection.

But patients with chronic fatigue often disapprove when this recommendation is made. "You're telling me it's all in my head," they say. But if a doctor believes this, that the patient has pathology "in his head," the treatment won't be up to standard. The attitude ought to be that, when someone suffers chronic tiredness without physical cause, further thinking — a lot of further thinking — is in order. That's what psychotherapy is. It's today's way of thinking about things with a doctor, things like chronic fatigue syndrome included. It's also the way to approach fibromyalgia, multiple personality disorder, and multiple chemical sensitivities. Although some who suffer in these ways will be offended, it's indisputable that, since we know of no causes for these states, much more thinking — psychotherapy usually — is in order.

✤✤✤

Mr. Yang Keyuan, a researcher at a local drug company, was my patient twenty-five years ago. Obviously depressed, he'd come to my office with physical complaints, headaches, and general unwellness, which was a bit strange, because he knew I was a psychiatrist. A good scientist, he'd expected a pill, and was uneasy when I asked about his life. What sticks in my mind was his father, a high-ranking officer in the pre-Maoist Nationalist army. Both parents were linked to Chiang Kai-shek, part of the generalissimo's glamorous social circle. After the unexpected arrest and execution of his father by Chiang Kai-shek, his mother and the rest of the family continued as members of the inner circle. Only after he'd graduated from college did Mr. Keyuan move to Canada.

"How did you feel about your mother's continued association with Chiang Kai-shek after your father was executed?" I asked.

The question had never crossed Mr. Keyuan's mind. Disconcerted, he cut short our meeting, but did agree to come for a second appointment, which, a few days later, he cancelled. It took several weeks before he got up the nerve to set up a regular schedule. We met twice a week for a year. He turned out to be not only intelligent, but psychologically sophisticated and creative. When he stopped coming, he felt the psychotherapy had been a big help.

Today, so many years later, I understand better what was going on. Then, short on cultural sophistication, I had judgemental thoughts like, *Is his denial ever intense!* and, *He's so intellectually sophisticated, yet using primitive defence mechanisms.* What I didn't understand was that, being Chinese, psychological reflection wasn't his first choice as a way to address such troubles. To most Asians, Western psychologizing isn't the fashion; the Western version of introspection is typically considered to be navel-gazing. Focusing on the body is much preferred. That's why, in Asia, neurasthenia is the diagnosis given to those we call depressed. It's also why, when choosing placebos, Asians generally prefer herbs and Westerners prefer psychotherapy.

Every culture has a symptom pool. It is acceptable and common for a Canadian to select symptoms like depression and headache, whereas in Malaysia it is common to fear one's penis is shrinking up into the body. Explanations of the reasons for psychiatric disease are also culturally embedded. In France, the tendency is to attribute chronic fatigue syndrome to educational practices; in Scandinavia, leakage from the amalgam fillings in our teeth is more often implicated; the commonest American suspicion is that it's caused by viral infections. Mr. Keyuan had picked neurasthenia, a symptom from the Chinese symptom pool, one that was previously available for Westerners but is currently outmoded; but he's also Westernized, so he visited a talking doctor.

In the past twenty-two years, Mr. Keyuan and I have had lunch twice. The last time, he told a story: When someone at home has a fishbone in his throat, he takes a bowl of water, faces east, and, with his free hand, traces a secret Chinese character on the surface of the water. This is not an officially known character, but resembles that for a dragon. The afflicted person drinks the water, and in a few hours the bony dilemma is resolved. Mr. Keyuan is a scientist, and when he saw my faint smile, responded with a faint smile of his own. Long Westernized, he'd already gone through the pain of weakening cultural traditions, that is to say, the fading of his once-preferred superstitions. Just the same, and again with a smile, he once showed me a small bottle he carried with him at all times. It contained a liquid which he said would cure the cough of which I had complained. Its label read:

PO SUM ON
Peppermint Oil, 57.30 ml.
Dragon Blood, 2.07 gm.
Cinnamon Oil, 0.96 ml.
Species of Skullcap, 0.58 gm.
Liquorice, 0.32 gm.
Tea Oil, 100 ml.

Traditions and superstitions, invisible in one's native culture, are corrupted in new surroundings: like radioactive isotopes, placebo cures have a half-life. When asked to rethink our own traditions, we're surprised, because to us they'd always been invisible. Supported by our own culture — newspapers, television, journals, public opinion — Western doctors, invited to notice and change our own ceremonial practices, such as placebo traditions, for example, are faced with a far greater wrench than Mr. Keyuan.

✢ ✢ ✢

Although Prozac exploits the common belief that swallowing things cures health problems, there are many psychiatric methods, some still in use, that at first glance don't suggest they could be helpful. Psychiatric zealots once administered insulin-coma treatments to those called schizophrenic and performed pre-frontal lobotomies (an instrument was used to puncture the upper part of the eye socket, then pushed into the frontal lobe of the brain; this was later done with more sophisticated instruments). These procedures proved useless. An important point is that, although at first primitive, attempts were made to render these procedures humane.

I myself gave electroshock treatments as a student, at that time done crudely. Strong attendants held the arms and legs of the patient so he wouldn't injure himself. I pressed the button on the machine to send the electric current through the brain, which induced a grand-mal convulsion. I didn't see it myself, but knew that sometimes bones were fractured by the power of the convulsion.

We, too, tried to make the procedure more humane. That year (I was in my first year of training), the procedure was changed. Just before the current was passed through the patient's brain, a muscle-paralyzing drug, Anectine, was injected intravenously. In the two or three seconds between the injection and the unconsciousness brought on by the electric current, these patients were paralyzed, unable to move, breathe, or cough. Albeit briefly, the sensation was frightening and unpleasant. The important point is that this protected patients from fracturing their bones; a humane practice had been added. Nowadays, many newer humane practices have been added: full anesthesia to eliminate the unpleasant fear that goes along with paralysis; newer electric currents that cause less memory loss; currents applied to specific parts of the brain, also with the effect of decreasing complications.

Current psychiatric rhetoric is that electroshock treatment plays a valuable role in the treatment of depression, and, to a lesser extent, in the treatment of schizophrenia. Yet no one knows whether this is or is not a placebo effect. Apart from my despair that my colleagues give little thought to placebos, I'm not concerned about electroshock; it's now virtually without side effects. My chief concern is different: unless the patient wants it, why should *any* "treatment" be given to those who have no sense of themselves as sick? That the patient agrees to a treatment, usually after strong persuasion by doctors and family, is beside the point.

You can see what I'm suggesting: all human actions are culture bound — rituals, in other words. Although many will find this hard to swallow, there are no acts that are without a cultural referent or pattern. The only human actions *not* culture bound are those performed due to indisputable physiological causes: sweating, secretions in the nose, blood circulation. The only *abnormal* human actions that are not culture bound are those due to physiological abnormality: tremors, paralyses, spasms, wasting (those that occur in the presence of disease or injury, in other words). We don't even call such things human actions. So, in the absence of disease, we're led straight to culture.

Drawing attention to precious group beliefs, even pointing out blatantly faulty logic, has little effect. Groupthink is powerful, even among those who want to be scientific. We can't live without caucus solidarity, but once they are institutionalized, bad habits are hard to shed.

Some rituals have short lives and quickly fade. I don't know whether psychiatrists still tell patients to strap lights to their heads — the idea was that fewer hours of light in the winter causes depression — but I don't hear about it nowadays. Because lots of us, me included, find it silly, this practice didn't fit into our culture well and therefore has had weak staying power. But snake oil (snakes bottled up in wine) in South-east Asia, and copper bracelets in the West — both supposedly effective for arthritis — have lasted a long time.

❖ ❖ ❖

I'm unsure, but suspect the antidepressant craze will fade. For years, antidepressants were magically effective, and it was popular to tell stories of patients who, before Prozac, had long, futile careers as psychotherapy patients. Then, when given Prozac, presto, they were cured. Stubborn skeptic, I kept doing my version of psychotherapy. Because most of my patients got better quickly, some almost instantaneously, I was enthralled by my own presto cures. I made jokes about this: patients who get better in psychotherapy, I said, have experienced the Prozac effect; those who get better on Prozac have experienced the psychotherapy effect.

Dr. David Healy, a Welch psychiatrist and expert in antidepressants and the history of psychopharmacology, reports that selective serotonin re-uptake inhibitors (SSRIS), the group of antidepressants of which Prozac is a member, are not available in Japan;[10] in that culture, they haven't found themselves a place. The Western epidemic of depression didn't happen in Japan. Instead, people take anxiolytics — tranquilizers like Valium. There's something fishy here, something about cultural fashions in psychiatric illness. It suggests we haven't paid attention to what counts as real evidence.

Although, as mentioned earlier, the difference between them and placebos is slight, clinical trials convince psychiatrists that antidepressants are effective. But the effect, if there is one, is minimal; the results of really effective treatments are so obvious that no clinical trials are needed. Penicillin eliminated brain syphilis so quickly and effectively that it would have been preposterous to subject it to clinical trials. Insulin given to a diabetic patient works even faster; within minutes, a patient with diabetic acidosis is cured. And the anesthetic pentothal, injected, instantly induces sleep. When there are many treatments for the same disorder — depression is treated with drugs, electroshock, and psychotherapy — doctors other than psychiatrists assume no definitive treatment has yet been found. In psychiatry, there is an even more fundamental reason to worry about this: no *disease* has been found.

How is it that we give scientific status to obviously shamanic cures? I'm more amazed than ever when people swear allegiance to things that are nothing more than ideas. Freud, Adler, Jung, yogic flying, and Deepak Chopra have followers galore, as do Prozac and psychiatric biology. Some of these ideas are intriguing, but all are *poetic* ideas, unfortunately put forward sincerely and earnestly. As Oscar Wilde once said, "All bad poetry is sincere." As often as not, these ideas attract interest from people according to the social group to which they belong. I'm impressed by the ideas of Freud, someone else by the ideas of Deepak Chopra. Because he uses technical words, it's obvious some will think Freud's poetry is bad. Such attitudes are, so to speak, class-related.

Those, for example, who read *The New York Review of Books* think Deepak Chopra's poetry is bad. But on Judgement Day it will be declared that Freud, Adler, Jung, yogic flying, and Deepak Chopra are to be found both interesting and harmless.

Prozac and psychiatric biology, bad poetry indeed, are *not* harmless. But don't worry. Drug side effects on the one hand, and the belief in biological inferiority on the other, guarantee they won't have the staying power of Shakespeare.

Led off track by their allegiance to blind empiricism, psychiatrists who don't understand about the placebo effect treat anxiety with everything that comes to hand: cognitive behaviour therapy, interpersonal therapy, psychoanalysis, empathy, desensitization, benzodiazepines, antidepressants — even with neuroleptics (antipsychotic drugs). It's important to note that they also use this cornucopia of methods to treat every other psychiatric disorder: schizophrenia, mania, personality disorders, depression, geriatric patients, traumatized patients, and culturally diverse populations. This is peculiar, because in medicine it is expected that each disease has a specific treatment.

All of these methods "work" for all disorders, yet no one is amazed. But there *are* official criteria for their use — this year. Students, to pass their exams, must know the treatments currently favoured. Next year the exam answer will be different.

I'm either grandiose or old-fashioned — or simply have my head screwed on right. Since I'm a specialist, it seems obvious I've been assigned the job of working with any psychiatric misery that comes my way. What good doctors say to their patients isn't in a book, a manual, or a theory; the topic is dictated by what our patients talk about.

Despite increasing medical reports that cast doubt on the effectiveness of antidepressant drugs, depression has become an epidemic, mostly because doctors are diagnosing it right, left, and centre. Almost every person who comes to my psychiatric outpatient clinic these days announces himself by saying he is depressed. That modern depression has qualities of a communal hysteria has implications that could upgrade psychiatric thinking; the suggestion that mimesis (imitation, mimicry) might be central to depression bears serious consideration.

In his book *Mourning and Melancholia*,[II] Freud gave many illustrations of how the depressed adopt the self-insulting actions, thoughts, and attitudes of other important people in their lives.

I have no doubt that the most promising explanations of human behaviour consider mimesis to be central. Indeed, the area in the brain that represents imitation — identification, mimicry, mimesis — is even larger than that for language. The tendency to identify with our parents, our community, and our country is easy to see; identifying with important cultural archetypes lies at the heart of all human acts. Homosexuality, revolution, conformism, artistry, being a warrior, and becoming a doctor all require a model. Even trivial actions — how one acts on the subway train, the manner in which one enquires at an information booth — are fraught, laden with culturally informed elements.

✤ ✤ ✤

The key point is that superstition — communal belief — is the wonderful underpinning of human life; the *accusation* of superstition is the darker side of human life. It gives away our eternal caste systems: worshippers at a Voodoo shrine are untouchables, our inferiors, superstitious. We, of course, are Brahmins.

Arrogantly, most save the word "superstition" for unfamiliar practices, what *others* do. What *we* do makes sense. Therefore, when I try to make placebo ceremonies visible, I often use exotic examples, my intent being always to say, "We do this, too, but in a way that, to us, stays invisible."

The word "ceremony" is most commonly attached to rituals performed in religious institutions, especially rituals sanctified by a long history and ardently believed in; the word "treatment" gets attached to rituals sanctified by being performed in medical or healing centres. Confusion arises because doctors, as well as unwittingly delivering medical rituals — placebo cures — can cure real physiological diseases. The important point is that we're all superstitious and ready to believe blindly. When we deride religious practices we need to think again.

We don't see that having a sore knee rinsed out and its frayed cartilage trimmed is a superstition, because we believe it helps and makes sense. But it's now known the pain reduction it produces is a placebo effect. When I said this to a friend who's had his knee rinsed-and-trimmed, I was rewarded with howls. It reminded me of telling a health-food aficionado that artificial sweetener, whisky, and staying up late are not problems. In certain cultural sub-communities (the one I live in), debridement and lavage of the knee joint is believed in.

Here's an example of "science" and the logic that follows from it: those who smoke have become addicted to the chemical nicotine, addiction meaning the body has developed a physiological need for nicotine. That's why it's hard to stop smoking. Those who wish to stop will be helped by taking small doses of nicotine by mouth or by using a nicotine patch to tide them over as they undergo withdrawal from nicotine.

This is logical, right? In line with medical science, right? But it's wrong. In the strict sense of the word, nicotine is not very addicting. It's socially compelling (note that smoking is an excellent example of mimesis), and highly rewarding — perhaps. But to the chagrin of many who read these words, it's mostly a habit. Although smokers are powerfully habituated to smoking, and enjoy it very much, when compared to physiological addictions (to narcotics, cocaine, barbiturates, amphetamines, and, for heavy users, alcohol), the addiction to tobacco is weak. A scientific frame has been applied illogically.

Those with strong physiological addictions — to barbiturates, amphetamines, heroin, cocaine — aren't just habituated to their drugs; they are physiologically dependent and get physically sick when the drug they are addicted to isn't available. Rats and mice like nicotine — but it's not an addiction. They don't get sick if cut off. Even for bona fide addicts — those who are hooked on heroin and cocaine — the habituation is more powerful than the addiction; after getting off drugs, addicts often go back to them. They get over the addiction, but the habit — the habituation — is alive and well. That's why alcoholics who haven't had a drink for years repeat their well-known mantra that they *are* alcoholics, not that they *were* alcoholics. And that's also why, thirty-five years after I stopped, I still take the occasional drag on an imaginary cigarette.

The primary issue for a drug addict is his sense of who he is: "I'm the guy who takes this or that drug, is part of this or that social group, lives this or that sort of life." Because the self-defining habit is in the addict's head, I like to classify it as a personally designed placebo, an unusual use of the term placebo but a usage to which I'm trying to habituate anyone who listens. Taking drugs and belonging to a drug culture is, for addicts, a ceremonial activity that sets straight for him who he is; he's one thing but not another, the one who shoots up, pops uppers and downers, and isn't one of the conventional, clean, and conformist dorks.

It's important to notice how deeply attached we are to theories like smoking being a true addiction to nicotine, an attachment that is quite different from the cool impersonality of *real* scientific findings. I say this because both anti-smoking campaigners and friends who smoke will be annoyed at what I've said. They insist that smoking is a "real" addiction. Few of my ex-smoker friends are histrionic, but a sub-group of anti-smoking campaigners, very histrionic indeed, will be outraged when they read my argument. "Of course it's an addiction," they'll say. "Medical science has proved that . . ." But it hasn't. In other words, placebo cures for smoking, whether in patches, lozenges, chewing gum, or pills, aren't used because of idle gullibility; like all types of communal passion they are passionately believed in and held on to.

Were someone diagnosed as suffering from pneumococcal pneumonia and I said, "Listen, I don't think there's any such thing as pneumococcal pneumonia," the response would be calm and mildly surprised.

"Really," I would be told. "Didn't you study bacteriology? Remember when we were medical students, we looked at the bacteria in the sputum and in the slides of lung tissue? We cultured the bacteria on agar plates and tested them for sensitivity to antibiotics."

But if I say, "Hey, I don't think there's such a thing as fibromyalgia (or chronic fatigue syndrome, learning disability, schizophrenia, et cetera)," there is outrage. Doctors have conditioned unhappy people to think they have diseases and, once popularized, the idea isn't to be questioned. Once I join in on the medical dislike of naturopaths, it's hard to change my mind. Since other doctors share my skepticism, I'm supported and encouraged to carry on with my belief.

"What do you mean?" I'll be told when I doubt the high incidence of depression. "Don't you know that hundreds of doctors believe in it, that it's been shown that it's caused by . . ."

Such protestations lead Shakespeare to prompt me: "The lady doth protest too much, methinks." Hamlet said this wistfully, as wistfully as doctors, who, knowing they are speaking with unhappy, ill persons, understand that they mustn't voice their doubts blatantly. The offended sufferer will go on and on, call on opinions, web sites, and organizations (propaganda groups), but will never point to scientific evidence. The sentence "It's been shown that it's caused by . . ." won't be completed. The interesting thing to me is the emotional outrage, which doesn't happen if I'm skeptical about a disease that really exists. In that case, the response is measured, perhaps puzzled, and produces real information about the disorder. No one is uncompromising about biological facts; fanaticism is reserved for mysteries, such as the shroud of Turin, the final Utopia, what Freud really meant.

If I say someone is crazy, everyone knows what I mean; it's a good Middle English word, solidly grounded in everyday use. We "get" the meaning of the word because of its "clang" effect: it resonates deeply. The usual response is, "Oh, yeah, I know what you mean. He's crazy." The word puts across an idea that, although clear, also refers to a familiar category of behaviours, and — most important — doesn't commit us to final conclusions.

If I say someone is schizophrenic, I have become melodramatic about a common way of life, ominous-sounding because of its Greek roots, one that leads to worry and bewilderment. But there's no echo in the soul. The response it evokes is different to what happens if we're told someone is "crazy." "What is schizophrenia, anyway?" is what people ask me. That existential question is a trap, one that doctors, me included, are always at risk of falling into, thinking we're identifying something real — "schizophrenia" — when we're only pointing at a disturbing style of human behaviour.

There is no end to arguments and explanations, popular until a new fiction comes along to take its place. But psychiatry isn't prone to give up its fictions; madness is so bothersome we fear giving up received ideas. Safely slotted into the bad-brain, bad-chemical theories, we heave a sigh of relief. However, since severe madness is the centre-piece of psychiatric work, this misunderstanding of madness pollutes our understanding of all patients. Gradually, every misery is suspect: it's biological. Remembering the truth — that we have no explanations for madness — immunizes us.

✤ ✤ ✤

As a pediatric resident in 1960, I worked for a month for Bill Mustard, an acclaimed heart surgeon. Because he was known to be hard on residents, I was nervous, and since he knew I was planning to train as a psychiatrist, I figured I'd be goaded and teased more than most. Yet he never tormented me.

It was said that, before operations, he never saw the young children upon whom he was to operate; his senior resident and the referring doctor did that part. Already a psychiatrist in my mind, I figured he was a tough surgeon trying to hide his soft and sentimental side, a man who couldn't face a real child who, the next day, might die. Bill Mustard was the perfect example of the technological doctor; I'm the perfect example of the aesthetic doctor. He corrected tangible maladies; I deal with fire and air.

But Mustard and I aren't the opposite extremes we appear to be on the surface. Underneath, he was a sentimentalist, and I, arguing on behalf of aestheticism and hysteria, am a tough realist. The ancient Greeks thought the gods governed all their actions. At the same time, they knew that they themselves were the ones who swung an axe at an enemy, made a sacrifice, and embraced their wives. In other words, like Bill Mustard and me, they indulged in doublethink.

Doublethink is universal: my wife, an angel, is a pain in the neck; I want to write my five hundred words today, and, it's stupid to be a work fanatic; the church in which I grew up awes and inspires me, and, the church I grew up in is a boring orthodoxy. Logicians and rationalists, on the other hand, think they can get to a single truth, one free of superstition and doublethink, and have therefore escaped superstition. But only uninformed scientists think they discover the truth. In the long run, all theories break down, although along the way, they may have practical value. Theories never announce the truth.

CHAPTER THREE

DRUGS VERSUS PLACEBOS

IT'S EASY TO DESCRIBE PLACEBO CURES FROM history, from popular culture, and from anthropology, descriptions of treatments that yield results as promising and convincing as anything we psychiatrists have come up with. It isn't that science is flawed; it's that most psychiatric research isn't scientific. Instead, researchers rely on a show of hands — surveys, opinion polls — to which they attach scientific-sounding words. All articles in psychiatric journals document their cures and improvements by recording the results of patients' opinions. No psychiatric article exists that documents cures by way of objective evidence. Anyone, especially any real scientist, understands the necessity of objective evidence.

Because I'm out to make people think differently about madness, neurosis, and every other human folly, I use certain words in new ways — sometimes surprising and provocative ways. Since the power of the placebo is my main prop as I undermine current psychiatric methods, its power must be fully appreciated, so I don't limit myself to talking about the sugar pills we doctors once gave to nervous patients. Nor do

I refer only to the sugar pills used as comparison medications when new drugs are tested.

The word "placebo," I'm arguing, can to be applied to all human behaviours and styles of life. In other words, every choice of how we should live has as its aim to be self-comforting, seems at the time to be our best current option, intends to make life better — to heal our souls. Other choices have been shunned because they are unattractive or disturbing.

This model can be used to explain why, without good reason, psychiatrists cling so urgently to their disease and treatment theories. Obviously, they *prefer* to believe in these theories, and although this preference gives them comfort, it also steers them away from points of view they don't want to know about, views that are odd or unsettling. They are sick at heart, I assume, about seeing their patients' fears, suffering, and madness for what they are, and cure this state with two words: disease and treatment. These words are their own placebo, a metaphoric treatment for a metaphoric sickness.

Being reborn in Christ, finding the girl of your dreams, or changing the direction of your life in accord with astrological prediction can also cure the sick-at-heart. Once I've worked with them psychoanalytically, my patients are cured, too. But of what could I be curing them? As far as I can tell they suffer from the same idiocy, decency, and ecstasy as I do.

When unfamiliar, placebos are brilliantly visible; alien placebos look odd. When they appear in foreign cultures we call them superstitions. When they become visible in our own we say that, unfortunately, a few remnants of superstition endure, a stubbornly persistent rump of silliness of which we must, and soon will, rid ourselves.

Blithely, in the fifth century, Herodotus anticipated modern smugness. He wrote of his amazement at how simple-minded people had been a hundred years earlier, especially in comparison to the Greeks of his time, who, he said confidently, were shrewd and free of superstition. Dressed up as science, our own placebos — superstitions — are equally invisible to us. But Goethe reminds us in *Maximen and Reflexionen* that, "Superstition is the poetry of life."

✢ ✢ ✢

Nowadays, almost every patient who comes to my clinic says he's depressed. I'm not the first to notice that psychiatric symptoms are subject to fashion, and because a *real* disease wouldn't change its symptoms, it's important to notice this. That patients once complained less often of depression, preferring compulsions, obsessions, and relationship problems, disappoints anyone who wants to believe that they are real diseases. It's amazing that one man raves in the fashion of another who came before him; the symptoms of ecstatics and madmen are, like the symptoms of the rest of us, not independent creations; they're learned by rote from their surroundings. Though symptoms are adopted from history and from culture, they also differ according to the era in which they appear.

We have wonderful drugs for the treatment of depression, say the colleagues who think their patients are somatically abnormal, an idea that excites them so much they haven't noticed that the incidence of depression exploded as soon as it was thought there was a drug treatment available. I'm pretty sure that, more often than not, these excellent outcomes of treatment are yet another placebo effect. An unsettling angle on this is that the promotion of antidepressants, originally developed as anti-anxiety drugs, has been part of a marketing strategy.

Everyone knows countless antidepressive tricks, rivals to Prozac, and often more effective. Most of us have experimented with them: falling in love, religion, finding someone to blame, buying a house, getting divorced. Workaholic doctors, researchers, and inventors cure themselves through industry, and artists madly paint, write, and compose. For still others, daring sexual antics are the *sine qua non* of antidepressive success.

David Healy (whom I mentioned briefly in Chapter 2) points out in his fine book *The Antidepressant Era*[1] that, in 1987, Prozac (fluoxetine) was licensed on the basis of its minimal superiority over placebo — and its *inferiority* to the drug gold standard, Tofranil (imipramine), a medication still in use. Prozac was not shown to have beneficial effects for hospitalized patients. Even its mildly helpful effect with outpatients was suspect, because so many non-hospitalized patients take other drugs as well, most commonly drugs from the Valium family. And of Tofranil, we can only say with certainty that it's a good tonic. Its antidepressant effects are less clear.

Publicizing this information makes it easy to become the bearer of unpopular news: saying the effects of these drugs are minimal or non-existent reaps a bitter harvest. Because many people have been helped by antidepressants, I'm bound to cause embarrassment, mostly because people will think I'm saying, "The beneficial effect of these pills is all in your head." Of course these effects are psychological, but the phrase "in your head" is an accusation, an insult. However, there is nothing new or surprising about responding to inert treatments because it has been suggested that they will help.

Medieval tricksters, for example, travelled the countryside offering to cure the mad by removing a contaminating agent: a stone of folly lodged in the brain. These proto-psychiatrists opened the skull and removed the offending stone. They didn't, of course, actually trepan the skull. A cut in the scalp, some blood, and sleight of hand were the only requirements. Colleagues in Africa sucked out an evil spirit, then spit it into their palm in the form of a bloody worm — or a rolled-up bit of fluff that had been under the tongue, bloodied by biting the cheek.

Strangely, a moment's thought makes it clear that these "primitive" practitioners were more scientific than those who now prescribe anti-depressants. A healer who extracted the stone of folly or demonstrated a bloody worm that's been sucked out of a belly was a trickster, clear about what he'd done, but he wasn't foolish; he knew it was a conjuring trick. In contrast, when doctors treat depression and fibromyalgia as though they are real diseases, they believe in their ceremony as much as their patients do. They are full participants in a medical hysteria.

Were we observed by natives of Papua New Guinea, Western psychi-atric methods would look just as exotic as tribal cures. Electric currents passed through people's brains? Light contraptions strapped to their heads? People lying on couches and talking into the air (my patients, in other words)? And pills galore. Students raise their eyebrows when they hear that my patients lie on my couch, but they don't react scornfully.

These are Western rituals, and they don't look ridiculous to us. Nor do they provoke in us the "how superstitious we are!" reaction.

There was a time when all doctors were in the same boat, for up to a hundred years ago, almost all medical treatments were placebos. Bloodletting, ardently believed in for centuries, is a good example to keep in mind, as is sanatorium treatment for tuberculosis. Hundreds of thousands spent their life savings on a treatment whose rationale was unfounded. It's instructive to read Thomas Mann's Nobel Prize–winning novel, *The Magic Mountain;*[2] the rituals of sanatorium treatment are dignified, comforting, and disturbing.

I suspect that real, medical-technologic advances are precisely what forced modern psychiatry into existence. People want and need the magic gestures of doctors, and psychiatrists, even though they don't seem to know it, are now the only doctors who are single-minded about having such gestures on offer.

✢ ✢ ✢

Drug companies who lure doctors into using their products know the limitations of their studies, publicize them selectively and cleverly, and manipulate doctors into believing their inflated claims. In this relationship, doctors are credulous clients, naive believers, and the placebo effect of the drugs reassures them that they have a treatment available. We aren't the first to be credulous about depression. In 1621, Robert Burton wrote in *The Anatomy of Melancholy*[3] that it was clear what needed to be done:

> For melancholy, take a ram's head that never meddled with a ewe . . . boil it well, skin and wool together . . . take out the brains, and put these spices to it, cinnamon, ginger, nutmeg, cloves. . . . It may be eaten with bread in an egg or broth.

✢ ✢ ✢

In October of 1994 there was a demonstration in Jefferson Square in front of the Louisville, Kentucky, courthouse. The "Prozac Trial," the action against the Eli Lilly pharmaceutical house, was taking place.[4] Scores of people, all carrying candles, were demonstrating, because they feared that, were the case lost, their Prozac would be taken from them. This is mass hysteria, the kind of cultural movement that, when pushing its agenda, confounds every attempt to learn whether drugs like Prozac have any antidepressant effect at all.

The doctors of whom I'm complaining are hurt and shamed when this point is pressed. They think that, when I talk about a placebo effect, I mean trickery or the foolishness of a gullible patient. But that's not the point: the placebo effect is not foolishness, nor is the doctor who creates the placebo effect a trickster. The study of placebos is almost certainly the most important topic psychiatrists can study, yet it's a research effort totally neglected. Prevailing attitudes damn cere-monial treatments as sops given to silence patients' complaints. The placebo effect is also a nuisance, say the researchers, a glitch that messes up their attempts to conduct error-free studies.

Patients are quick to believe a real, causal "thing" has made them better, including, for example, a religious intervention that may have pre-ceded the cure: God gets the credit. Nowadays, much of the Western world has been converted to a different religion: science. Except what they have placed on their altar isn't science, it's scientism — the excessive belief in the power of scientific knowledge and techniques. Science says, "Suspend belief, accept nothing as true, just observe and think," but this is hard to do. Many of us falter and cling to science as something to believe in. Sadly, those who long to find a place to plant their feet find the rules intolerable, stick out their chins, and defiantly believe.

We humans like simplicity, and hence fall into the trap of dreaming up causes. Since symbols are fuzzy and hard to nail down, doctors get nervous, and doubt symbols are potent enough to cause — and cure — diseases. The most nervous of all are psychiatrists, the ones who should be most familiar with the power of symbols. They hate the idea that their patients don't have diseases but are struggling with critically important symbolic dilemmas.

Why are so many doctors, especially newly trained psychiatrists, uneasy about noting that we live in symbolic worlds? "Goodness," they are liable to say, "you're saying we cure by using magic." Although "magic" is an important and evocative metaphor, one that I like, they aren't quite right. Why are they frightened of magic? After all, mystery is characteristic of human life and a potent medical attitude. If patients did not believe doctors are potent and wise — it's not a fact, it's an idea embedded in our culture — they wouldn't allow us to hear their secrets, inspect their nakedness, or enter their bodies with instruments or surgery.

Even the great riddle, schizophrenia, is as wonderfully enigmatic as ever. I know I'm supposed to say we are on the verge of discovering abnormal chemicals or synapses in the brain, but we're not, and enthusiastic colleagues who think they'll soon find causes for these unhappy ways of life are indulging in wishful thinking.

It's vital that we be clear about the distinction between reliability and validity. Even if we have reliable criteria for identifying a group of people who we would say have schizophrenia — and there's no reason why we can't — this says nothing about whether we've identified a valid disease. All of us have criteria for reliably identifying bullies, biological psychiatrists, and fundamentalist Christians, but this doesn't mean we've identified valid disease categories.

Chronic fatigue syndrome, multiple chemical allergies, and attention deficit disorder, although we can reliably identify those said to suffer from them, are questionable disease categories, as is schizophrenia. The first three are commonly understood as signs of unhappiness, ways in which patients let us know things are amiss. Those called schizophrenic aren't afforded this courtesy. They are assigned without question to the category of abnormal biology.

I wish I could make the questionable disease categories I've just mentioned — there are more — vanish, but this is an impossible, probably silly, hope. Since I'm a psychiatrist, I worry especially about diagnoses in my field, every one of which is dubious and liable to abuse. It doesn't seem to occur to biological psychiatrists that tossing out the unproven idea that psychiatric disorders have genetic causes suggests to patients that they are biologically inferior to the rest of us. Since the *attitude* towards questionable diagnoses can change, I feel I have to direct heavy artillery against those who take them seriously.

When we face off, biological psychiatrists and I are liable to argue about whether pigs have wings; there are no solid facts available in our discipline that they or I can summon as evidence. Our squabbles, even if silly, are an important illustration of common ways people act, just as important as the actions of psychiatric patients, and as valuable as observing love, lust, desire, and envy in action. Due to their deification of science, marvellous human behaviours like psychiatrists quarrelling are ignored by the psychiatrists who currently have the loudest voices. For many of them, psychiatry has become the study of serotonin, genetics, and other topics they hope will demonstrate "bad" protoplasm.

When cornered, biological psychiatrists admit nothing has been discovered, which is no surprise because there is nothing to discover. Madness, as it should be, is an eternally troubling and amazing mystery, just as amazing as many other forms of human behaviour: criminality and nobility; enchantment by the ridiculous; commitment to the well-being of patients; artistry and genius; marital squabbling; tobacco addiction; falling in love. If we take note, everything we do is amazing. This doesn't mean psychiatrists don't offer help; it means only that human suffering is eternal, and psychiatrists will always practise their psychological methods, even if, at first, they don't seem as orthodox as other doctors.

⁘ ⁘ ⁘

The following examples have been assembled by art historian and broadcaster Simon Schama,[5] further confirmation that, in contrast to the familiar, the unfamiliar sounds foolish. It's the story of saints flocking back to Antwerp during the Counter-Reformation:

> St. Wilgefortis, whose flowing beard protected her against would-be violators but not against her pagan father, who had

her beheaded, whiskers and all . . . St. Clare of Montefalco, together with her attribute of the balance, to remind her devotees of the three balls, posthumously discovered within her body, each of which weighed as much as the other two combined, a mysterious affirmation of the indivisible Trinity . . . Maria, engaged in holy lactatio, smiling as she hosed sweet milk directly into the thirsty mouth of St. Bernard of Clairvaux . . .

Preposterous? But what about the (incomplete) list of available antidepressants I have before me? There are twenty-one of them, as numerous as the Counter-Reformation saints who rushed into Antwerp and, like saints, all effective. Blessed with important-sounding scientific names, they don't offend our ears as do corpse-residing balls that stand for the Trinity, but our comfort with these names stems from familiarity, from their current cultural prominence.

What, I wonder, do non-psychiatric medical colleagues think when they hear we have so many treatments for one disorder? There are many gastric-acid-inhibiting drugs, but if a new one is more effective, it replaces older drugs quickly; the first antidepressants, now forty years old, despite competition from countless new drugs on the market, are still in use.

Like saints, the following drugs, the class of antidepressants called NSRIS, nonselective monoamine re-uptake inhibitors (there are at least five other classes), differ from one another in their chemical structure and their side effects, but not in their alleged therapeutic effectiveness: amitriptyline, clomipramine, desipramine, doxepin, imipramine, maprotiline, nortriptyline, and trimipramine.

What's happened, of course, is that drug companies take a proven drug, change one molecule, and market it as a new product, thereby enjoying a new round of profits and a twenty-year extension of patent rights, the so-called "me-too" drugs. The former editor-in-chief of the *New England Journal of Medicine*, Marcia Angell, has exposed the sordid details in her book *The Truth About the Drug Companies.*[6] Because it is expensive and unpredictable, the pharmaceutical houses have little interest in innovative research and count on universities and the United States's National Institutes of Health to make the basic science discoveries. They are particularly skilled at pious pronouncements about the high cost of research and development (see Merrill Goozner's book *The $800 Million Pill*.)[7]

Studies on the beneficial effects of antidepressants are fatally flawed. David Healy, whose book *The Antidepressant Era* I've already mentioned, makes no bones about this. He directs our attention to the most widely used instrument in research on depression, the Hamilton Rating Scale for Depression (devised by Max Hamilton in 1960). Healy points out that:

> In a sense, there is an element of rabbits and hats to Hamilton's scale. Its items, which cover sleep and appetite, could not have been better designed to demonstrate the effects of tricyclic antidepressants like imipramine, which are somewhat sedative and appetite stimulant *even in people who are not depressed.* [my italics]

In other words, the scale incorrectly suggests that these drugs lead to a change in appetite or sleep habits because some depressive illness has been cured, but they actually lead to a change in the appetite and sleep habits of everyone. Right off the bat, 12 percent of what the scale measures has nothing to do with depression. What Healy doesn't tell us is that, because these scales depend on the patient telling us whether or not he's been helped, they will never give us the answers we want. What a patient says can never distinguish an actual change in a disease state from a placebo response. Without a laboratory test, an objective sign, the distinction between objective and placebo-induced improvements cannot be made.

Schizophrenic patients don't consider themselves unwell, so when we struggle to determine whether they've been helped, they cannot answer; statements about being helped or not helped don't apply. Instead, after we have "treated" them, we are the ones who make judgements about whether they are better. The key word here is "judgement," which is neither more nor less than a preference: we like their behaviour better after we've suppressed their earlier behaviour with drugs. Since "better" is simply something that's to our taste, we are on shaky ground scientifically.

These facts are difficult for psychiatric doctors to stomach, because the Hamilton scale is a *test*, in short supply in the world of psychiatry. "What kind of doctor am I if I have no tests?" thinks the psychiatrist.

The truth is that psychiatry has spurious tests in abundance; real ones don't exist. Despite centuries of trying, no psychiatric test that taps into objective evidence has ever been devised. Anything these tests do is done better by a good interviewer, hence they are used only by those who don't trust their own skills. Like an interview, questionnaires only tell how close a patient is to the average — how "non-unique" he is, in other words. Unless uniqueness, or deviation from the average, is correlated with a detectable — I stress *detectable* — piece of pathology, it means only that someone is odd or uncommon.

The best-known questionnaires are public-opinion polls. The only thing polls can predict is how respondents are likely to answer when polled again, hence projecting election results with fair accuracy. But people change their minds, a characteristic of patients who complete questionnaires as well as of voters.

I go further than Healy: I believe the whole scale is hogwash. The only thing a questionnaire can tell us is the patient's opinion, and an opinion is not a valid scientific datum. In the next chapter, I'll spell out why opinion has no value, and identify Robert Koch, the medical genius who laid out the scientific rules for what counts as a diagnostic sign of disease. A questionnaire requires a yes-or-no answer, a requirement that we obey the binary logic of computers. Diagnosis makes the same demand: patients either have a disease of they don't. Binary logic — either/or — must never replace the logic that works best for human matters: and/or, ambiguity, subtlety, and perhaps.

Healy goes on to explain that the other major depression scale used by researchers is equally flawed:

If there is an element of rabbits and hats to the Hamilton
scale, however, this is arguably no more than there has been
with its principal competitor, Beck's Depression Inventory
(BDI). The BDI focuses only on cognitive aspects of depression. It is difficult to imagine anyone who has been through
a cognitive therapy program not being biased toward
answering the particular items on the scale in a different
manner after therapy by virtue of the procedures of cognitive therapy, quite independently of any effect those
procedures may have on depressions. In the case of the BDI,
however, just as with the Hamilton scale, there has been a
group interested in accepting this scale: cognitive therapists. Another aspect of successful scales, then, is their need
to coincide with certain interests if they are to survive.

✣ ✣ ✣

What I've described is the tip of the iceberg; the flaws of biological
research are of minor importance, because they reflect only naïveté, a
human faculty common to enthusiasts keen on proving something.
The greater problem is that pharmaceutical houses must patent drugs
for a specific disease. Consequently, to survive, drug companies aim
their products at diseases, support research that targets diseases, and
influence psychiatric researchers to think in disease categories. Drug
companies cough up the money, and research becomes biased in the
direction of what pharmaceutical houses want.

If a product's patent expires, the drug companies simply designate
a new target and, to get a new patent, aim the same drug at a different
"disease." Because Prozac's patent expired in 2001, its price dropped
by 80 percent. The drug's manufacturer, Eli Lilly and Company,
stopped pouring money into promoting it as an antidepressant,
renamed it Sarafem, and repackaged in a lavender-and-pink capsule.
Because it has a new disease target, premenstrual dysphoric disorder,
it sports shiny new patent protection. It's obvious the diseases believed
in by the public and by naive psychiatrists are arbitrary categories

created for financial gain. In the service of good business, the humanity of those who are suffering is forgotten.

Is anyone surprised that drug companies make sure studies with positive outcomes are published several times and those with negative outcomes only once — if at all?[8] Certainly, if studies sponsored by drug houses are unfavourable, they don't get publicized. The mass favour found by drugs like Prozac is almost completely a result of drug-company propaganda and a placebo effect stirred up by gullible psychiatrists and occasionally by charlatans.

The role of drug companies is even more worrying if we ponder a catch-22: if a drug company does any research on the harmful side effects of a drug, it makes itself vulnerable to legal liability.

✤✤✤

In 1989, Joseph Wesbecker shot twenty of his co-workers in Louisville, Kentucky, killing eight. The manufacturer of Prozac, Eli Lilly of Indianapolis, became the target of a liability suit that alleged the drug had caused Mr. Wesbecker's murderous behaviour. John Cornwell's book *The Power to Harm*[9] documents the shocking story and, of particular interest here, the behaviour of the Eli Lilly company. According to Cornwell, during the trial the company flooded the media with information that discredited an important witness for the plaintiffs. Although the case against the pharmaceutical house failed, the presiding judge later published a motion stating his belief that Eli Lilly had secured this verdict with a secret payment to the plaintiffs. The amount was so large he characterized it as "mind-boggling." The judge claimed that in return for this payment, the plaintiffs had agreed to withhold evidence damaging to Eli Lilly's case.

I cringed when I read the testimony of the psychiatrists who gave evidence at the trial. I imagined what the lawyers on both sides might have thought: that the testifying scientists and doctors were being silly, making preposterous claims about drugs and human behaviour, desperately arguing the two sides of the nature/nurture issue.

✢ ✢ ✢

I'm uneasy about psychiatric drugs. Even those with valuable effects
— *especially* those with valuable effects — have serious side effects.
Some make patients feel odd, sometimes so odd that they feel like
zombies; they look and act like zombies, too. Neuroleptic drugs, the
drugs with which psychiatrists quiet psychotic patients (calm them?
subdue them?), make patients detached, an effect that is wonderful for
tranquilizing a psychiatric ward but liable to make a person, when
taking them, drive through red lights. Patients also become dependent
on some of these drugs, a state of "therapeutic drug dependency." In
other words, after taking them for a few months, to avoid withdrawal
symptoms (tardive dyskinesia), patients must take them forever.

Neuroleptics aren't like street drugs: they don't make us euphoric.
They will therefore never be saleable as street drugs. Some patients
take them willingly, but do so on rational grounds. While taking them,
they get important benefits: they stay out of hospital, can live with
family, and can keep jobs.

There is a body of literature that suggests that, except in the short
term, patients given neuroleptics ultimately don't do as well as those
not given them. The disturbing facts are in an article by Robert
Whitaker in *Medical Hypotheses*,[10] published in 2004. Robert Whitaker
is a journalist (a fine one, once a finalist for the Pulitzer Prize for a
science-related piece) and the author of *Mad in America*.[11] Many good
psychiatrists are aware of this article, but seem not to take it seriously.
Caught in the psychiatric culture, psychiatrists do what we all do
within our culture: carry on with our ways, even when we know our
ways are worrisome. Some common examples of this are smoking,
driving cars that consume too much fuel, and overeating, all of which
are in accord with common cultural habits.

If the results of treating the mad with these drugs are equivocal
enough to make such an article possible, we psychiatrists should at the
very least scratch our heads in bewilderment about what we've been
doing for fifty years. A strong response to this article would lead us to
instantly abandon the use of neuroleptic drugs.

Lithium and antipsychotic drugs definitely make manic and psychotic persons behave better, although we have to remember that "better" nearly always means their behaviour is better for us, we who are uncomfortable with manic or psychotic conduct. ("Quiet in the cellars; all the dogs nicely on their chains.") Manic and psychotic behaviour is especially awful for patients' families, so it may seem obvious that the more conventional behaviour inspired by these drugs is a good thing. Only some patients agree; many others feel they've been robbed of their own way of living and stop taking the drugs when unsupervised.

How much say, we must ask, do patients get in this matter? Although it's obvious medical treatment aims to reintegrate people into the social order, doctors dare not impose the social order they prefer. Unfortunately, psychiatric drugs, rather than restoring people to their place in the social order, have the potential to change the social order itself. Pimples, mischief, nervousness, oddity, imaginativeness, and wit are increasingly at risk of being under-represented.

The perturbing argument boils down to this: happiness is doing what most people do. So, if marriage is what most do, marry; if cell phones are popular, buy a cell phone; if coercing people to be conventional is customary, go along with it. In other words, psychiatrists, doing what most people do — being loyal to their peer group — give neuroleptic drugs to patients whose behaviour distresses us.

The value of psychiatric drugs is so obscured by the placebo effect that many of these patients can't be reasonably assessed at all. No one can predict which patients will show a placebo response, but statistics confirm what I've said. Best to say only that sometimes 30 and sometimes 90 percent of people show it, patients respond more powerfully to it the sicker they are, and dramatic treatments like surgery evoke it more strongly.

All assessments of drug effects are based on opinion, either the patient's or the doctor's, a wretched state of affairs, because opinions can't be separated from the opinion-giver's preference. You might think that, after drinking three martinis, my behaviour is vulgar; I might think it splendid, even after I've sobered up.

✣ ✣ ✣

I wouldn't be surprised if, a few years from now, antidepressant drugs suffer the same fate as insulin-coma treatment. In 1935, a Viennese psychiatrist, Manfred Sakel, thought he had discovered an amazing new treatment for schizophrenia. His patients, given large doses of insulin, had a high recovery rate. This is a remarkable claim, because schizophrenia is notoriously difficult to treat. Although the treatment eventually proved to be useless, it was in use for more than twenty years; I watched this treatment being given at the Queen Street Mental Health Centre in 1957. Every morning, a special group of patients was taken to a well-equipped suite of rooms, and given massive doses of insulin, massive enough to induce a deep coma. They were rigged up to intravenous equipment so that sugar could quickly be given if the coma became too deep. It was frightening to watch their noisy, restless breathing, knowing that the depth of the coma they were in verged on a point that might damage their brains.

The idea was that a deep regression of central-nervous-system functioning, followed by recovery, would allow for a healthier reintegration. This *seemed* to have an effect, both on patients and on the doctors who observed what happened, effects largely due to the drama of a risky "medical" treatment.

Hope springs eternal. When I was a psychiatric resident a few years later, similar methods were tried. Some of us were trained to induce regression in our patients by way of extreme isolation; others worked on units that used antipsychotic drugs in massive doses, trying to achieve the same regressive effect.

The idea of deep unconsciousness excites many of the heroic — and stupid — treatments that have been tried. Hypnosis, age regression, extreme isolation in a bare room, which was tried when I was a resident — all had the same mad rationale as the "New Age" regression to past lives, and similar to the nasty regression experiments funded by the CIA and carried out by Ewan Cameron at McGill University's Allan Memorial Institute, neatly disguised as scientific research.[12] These are rebirth fantasies, translated into quasi-medical language.

✦✦✦

Placebo cures tap into an array of cure images, our deeply held fantasies and beliefs. "Science" is the favoured code word. Doctors, herbalists, and chiropractors don't want to know that another word, "symbolism," is key. The acclaim we give the word science is what counts. But the "science" smokescreen is only a veil for the verbal magic that makes people feel better.

I've compiled a list of common methods for healing our souls — and many of our medical complaints. But it's only a list, and useful only if humility and reflectiveness are given a chance to wake it up. My list illustrates the common placebo approaches, all of which are gestures, messages, or signals. In other words, the healer is "speaking" in a coded language and saying two things: first, that he has the power and authority to do something; and second, that he has both an explanation of the illness and its cure. I've listed the common explanations given and believed in, although, since the number of placebo treatments is infinite, no list can be exhaustive.

- Cleansing and purifying oneself.
- Remembering and/or revealing a pathogenic secret (remembering an imagined harmful event from early childhood).
- Placing oneself in the hands of science, progress, or a powerful leader.
- Confessing and properly debasing oneself.
- Eating or swallowing some healing principle, or abstaining from eating and swallowing.
- Participating in a transformative ceremony or ritual.
- Scratching, cutting, or deforming one's body, including submitting to dramatic surgical procedures.
- Practising counter-magic (such as showing a cross to a demon to magically neutralize its magic powers).
- Receiving mystical emanations like hypnosis, psychic energy, undetectable X-rays, and electrical waves.
- Restoring one's lost soul or spirit.

+ Surrendering one's soul.
+ Moving the body in special ways, as in exercise, Tai Chi, and yoga.
+ Awakening and rebirth.

There are no essential game practices, said Wittgenstein. Some are played with balls, others with cards; still other games are played in the mind. Some require jumping, running, or skipping. And not all games involve winning, as we see with skiing, swimming, and playing catch. Wittgenstein is illustrating that games have in common only a family of resemblances, all vaguely related, by which we decide that the activity in question is a game. But there's no essence, no single, defining feature. There are only characteristics that overlap with those of other games.

That's the way ceremonial cures are recognized: there's a family relationship between ceremonial cures, but no essence; each involves several items from the above list.

Another characteristic of placebo cures is that they follow rules. I can't, for example, decide to cure myself by brushing my teeth. The culture has a system, a set of rules, about how we can be cured by cleansing, and it only works if I go along with the accepted ceremony. Exercise, enemas, laxatives, steam baths, and fasting all count as sanctioned cleansing ceremonies, which I can do alone, but which work better in a ceremonial setting like a health club, spa, or healer's office.

Usually, it's necessary to *believe* in the cure. But there are borderline cases. I, for example, feel better if I avoid sugar and drink my coffee with artificial sweetener, although I have no untoward reaction to sugar. This doesn't matter; I feel better, even though I know it does nothing. It's possible, of course, that I'm unconsciously indulging a *different* curative fantasy, one I secretly believe in, secret even from me. Perhaps, rather than purifying myself by avoiding sugar, I'm punishing myself, magically undoing my own gluttony.

+ + +

I, however, have bigger fish to fry. Ordinary minnows, day-to-day placebos, only hint at what I'm after; traditionally, obvious placebos aren't the only curative ceremonies. People get cured, find life more fulfilling, by actions that aren't thought of as treatments at all:

+ Affirming one's gender role, usually femaleness or maleness.
+ Seizing virtue and finding fault elsewhere.
+ Marrying and practising domestic life.
+ Seizing uniqueness, individuality, and self-reliance.
+ Becoming evil and committing crimes.
+ Enjoying humour.
+ Decorating or beautifying oneself.
+ Resorting to safe clichés, reductionism, and the misplaced use of aphorisms and slogans.
+ Gossiping.
+ Designing painful symptoms: craziness, depression, phobias, and every other psychiatric disorder.

The last of these, "every other psychiatric disorder," is a peculiar category, spectacularly interesting, but insofar as it's a cure that has to be cured, somewhat puzzling. But before spelling out why a "cure" needs to be cured, let me make a comment on my phrase "designing painful symptoms."

To say "designing" is to use a rhetorical trope, with which I aim to sting the mechanists now ascendant in psychiatry, the ones who misunderstand a statement by Descartes: "I have hitherto described this earth and generally the whole visible world, *as if it were* merely a machine in which there was nothing at all to consider except the shapes and motions of its parts" (my italics).[13] Descartes says "as if" because he understands the problem of taking metaphors literally, but, just the same, he slips into concretizing his metaphors. That's no big deal. As long as we are humble, are aware that every last one of us will mess up by taking metaphors literally, and remain vigilant about the use to which we put them, we can stay out of theoretical trouble. Richard Lewontin, an American evolutionary biologist at Harvard University, as keen to discount simple causality as I, puts it this way in his book *The Triple Helix:*[14]

The trouble with the general scheme of explanation contained in the metaphor of development is that it is bad biology. If we had the complete DNA sequence of an organism and unlimited computational power, we could not compute the organism, because the organism does not compute itself from its genes. Any computer that did as poor a job of computation as an organism does from its genetic 'program' would be immediately thrown into the trash and its manufacturer would be sued by the purchaser. Of course it is true that lions look different from lambs and chimps from humans because they have different genes, and a satisfactory explanation for the differences between lions, lambs, chimps, and us need not involve other causal factors. But if we want to know why two lambs are different from one another, a description of their genetic differences is insufficient and for some of their characteristics may even be irrelevant.

Naive mechanism has to be contradicted, so where many would say "happened," "developed," or "caused," and even though I know there is no inventor or designer, I stir things up by saying we "design," "create," and "invent" ourselves. I'm in good company; the ideology of biological mechanism is perfectly balanced by another ideology, the popular notion of self-expression and self-fulfillment. But just as no one can finger a biological cause or mechanism, there is no self that expresses or fulfills.

Psychiatric symptoms are solutions (a solution is a cure) to inner conflicts, compromises between the forces at play in every human life. These self-curative compromises, psychiatric symptoms, end up being treated by psychiatrists. In other words, psychiatric disorders and their accompanying symptoms are ways of life designed to make life bearable.

Symptoms are unpleasant self-portrayals. ("I'm the fearful, phobic man who can't manage any more and who needs to put himself into the hands of an authority figure, a doctor.") They keep at bay ideas judged to be even worse. ("I'm the guy who, by speaking English perfectly by the age of six, shamed and weakened my poor father who could hardly speak English at all. I therefore have to cancel this out. I do it by becoming fearful, phobic, and unable to manage.")

Symptoms solve something, and psychiatrists, agreeing that the solution is imperfect, try to help patients devise new solutions. Psychiatrists profit from the self-cures patients themselves have hit on. When we cure someone, we exploit his precious dreams and myths, his madness, solitude, and strangeness, the soothing personal tricks that buttress him against the fickleness of common life

✢ ✢ ✢

Yet emphasizing cures, superintelligence, and prolonged life suggests that we ought to dodge suffering, bewilderment, and tragedy completely. Desirable though health may be, because they can goad us into savouring what we've got, death and the unexpected aren't necessarily bad.

When I travel, as often as not I take a tour, immunized against full-blooded novelty. Although fun — a good place to watch oneself stake out a role in a group — a tour is also a glass cage, a piece of Canada, a *National Geographic* perusal of things in the company of people who, as often as not, already share my world. A tour gives the illusion that, although travelling, I'm also safe at home. Once, in Burma, alone and without itinerary, I was stressed — and awakened. When no one spoke English, I was unnerved, my eyes widened, I had no choice but to be part of Burma.

Perhaps in some Utopian world, as a way of achieving more awareness, every writer, psychiatrist, philosopher, judge, and politician would experience:

- Being in prison.
- Living in a shelter.
- Becoming a lunatic.
- Being under threat of death.
- Being hospitalized for a chronic illness.

+ Being raped.
+ Working in a sweat-shop.
+ Being on the receiving end of discrimination.

Finally there's my third list — the biggest fish and most ambitious cures we humans have occasion to seize on — the philosophies we live by:

+ Deep religious belief.
+ Paranoid battling against a world believed to be oppressive and persecuting.
+ Believing this to be the best of all possible worlds, a unrealistically optimistic conviction that life is sweet.
+ Believing deeply in rationality, progress, and science.
+ Skeptically finding everything meaningless.

As I tell about ceremonial cures — placebo cures of all sorts — you'll see they are underpinned by curative fantasies. As often as not, these fantasies can be found on my three lists.

CHAPTER FOUR

THE FALLACY OF SPECIFIC CAUSES

WE'RE DETERMINED, NOWADAYS, NOT TO SEE madness as a way of life, one of many kinds of cultural performance. We're committed to the idea that it's not a piece of our culture at all, it's medical abnormality. Although in the current psychiatric climate it's provocative to say so, I'm determined to show that madness is just another way of life, or, if you like, an odd and imaginative performance.

Although I doubt the psychiatric-disease idea, it's valuable to think about what we are up to when we take the disease idea seriously. Were it true, we'd be faced with a choice: is it insidious disquiet, imbalance, being out of sorts? Or is it specific, clear-cut, a malignant unknown that must be ferreted out, brought into focus, and tackled head on? In other words, are we to emulate Dionysus and the Romantics, approach madness speculatively, intuitively, and imaginatively, sensing only disharmony, or, in contrast, are we to be Apollonian, logical and incisive, and diligently search out specific causes?

These contrasting attitudes towards madness — indeed, towards the whole world — have a long and honourable history. Shakespeare portrayed Antony's dilemma in the same terms: should he succumb to Cleopatra's theatricality and dreaminess, her exotic voluptuousness, or should he be cunning, stand for reason and the well-being of the Roman Empire? Antony wasn't faced with a moral dilemma; his was the tragedy of being human, having to choose between, on the one hand, desire, joy, and beauty, and on the other, sobriety, conscientiousness, and getting things right. "I am fire and air; my other elements I give to baser life," said Cleopatra (V. ii. 289–290). Baser life means earth and water, the elements of good sense that are opposed to fire and air.

This is the secret theme of *Antony and Cleopatra*. Antony's marriage to Octavia is not impeded by his relationship with Cleopatra, because under Roman law Cleopatra has no legal status as a wife. Cleopatra, who lives according to the laws of love, finds it ludicrous that anyone would consider Antony to be married to Octavia. A spiritual husband, she says, easily trumps a legal husband.

Thomas Mann repeatedly acknowledged — and celebrated — these two ways of existing in the world: Life versus Mind. These are the approaches of Romance on the one hand, and of Enlightenment on the other. Psychiatrists wage the same battle, using our own language: pathology. We therefore distinguish hysterical enthusiasm and obsessive rationality as ways in which people approach the world. If I twist this question around upon ourselves, I can ask, In approaching madness, are psychiatrists best off being artists or logicians, hysterics or obsessives? Are psychiatrists fire and air, or are we earth and water?

✤ ✤ ✤

I'm talking about the muddle in which we doctors find ourselves, determined to cure diseases rationally but discovering that only now and then do our patients want such sport. Just as often they long for tonics, holistic health, and exotic flourishes. The best understanding of this dilemma comes by way of medical history.

The ancient idea was to figure out humoral imbalances, then correct them: achieve a proper balance of the four humours, which made up us all, blood (warm and moist), phlegm (cold and moist), yellow bile (warm and dry), and black bile (cold and dry). These four humours had many correlates: the four primary qualities (hot, dry, cold, and wet); the four seasons; the four ages of man (infancy, youth, adulthood, and old age); the four elements (fire, air, earth, and water); the four temperaments (sanguine, bilious, melancholic, and phlegmatic). Sometimes, in order to fine-tune the diagnosis, the permutations of the zodiac were correlated with humoral events. To modern ears this sounds silly, an ancient version of bioharmonics, cures by malarkey like tonics, ocean voyages, bloodletting, laxatives, and mountain air.

The valuable element in humoral conceptions of diagnosis and treatment is that it addresses the ordinary disquiet for which so many people visit their doctors. Conversations with such patients are coded, the exchanges symbolic: "You're out of sorts, and I understand it," the doctor says, or, "You're a physical and mental wreck, and I can help." As it has always been, being "out of sorts" or "a wreck" means your humours are out of whack.

Cures for humoral maladies, true to this day, are: a cold cloth on the forehead, plumping up the pillow, a darkened room, looking at the sufferer's tongue, advising a "mental-health day." These methods acknowledge illness, signal concern, and reassure; they are vital. But if gestures are vital, do rationalists like me have to reassess our scorn for acupuncture, herbal medicines, astrology, and homeopathy? It's clear the history of medicine before the nineteenth century was almost completely the history of placebos.

Just as, when the ancients said we are made up of earth, water, fire, and air, they forgot they were speaking in metaphors, so, during the two thousand years that humoral theory dominated medicine, doctors also forgot, becoming literal, concrete, and technical about ways of speech that are only poetic. We seem unable to stop confusing literal truth with metaphors, an epidemic malady from which we all suffer: *literalis terminalis*.

✢ ✢ ✢

Metaphor is a big word, more complicated than we were taught in elementary school: instead of saying things directly, we often use alternate words or phrases, clever analogies, or pictures. The greater truth about metaphors is that they are devices needed to grasp anything at all. If, for example, we want to use the strategy of objectivity to study something, we adopt the metaphor of "things" and "facts," objects that can be identified and studied, the usual stance used by science. If, instead, we use Cleopatra's metaphors of fire and ice, we can identify and study topics other than objects: romance, tragedy, love, and sex. Although it's common to try to study sex as an objective thing, Cleopatra was right: for sex, the metaphors of science don't work well.

Even the biological approach is a metaphor (it's actually a subcategory of the "objects" metaphor). The scientist says to himself, "Let's tackle human behaviour, using the metaphor of biology, and see whether it helps us out." That the biology metaphor hasn't come up with evidence that madness is a disease is important, but it's also important to keep in mind that all theoretical stances are tentative, experimental metaphors. That physics and chemistry have been spectacularly successful doesn't mean we've discovered the truth, only that, when we study things as objects, we've invented a really valuable metaphor. The dramatic successes of objective science mislead psychiatrists — and all doctors — making them hope they can discover physical causes for madness. "Physics envy," I call it. Like Lord Rutherford the New Zealand-born British Nobel laureate, they believe that all of science is either physics or stamp collecting. Physics explains, while other commentary is merely classification. This is amusing because psychiatry explains no diseases, but has authored the grotesque classification system called DSM-IV.

Thomas Szasz's *Myth of Mental Illness*,[1] first published in 1960, is the most comprehensive attack on psychiatry I know, harsh, uncompromising, and, insofar as he attacks the notion of mental disease, irrefutable. It is still in print. In reading the book today, I see that he uses arguments similar to mine. Since there are no diseases, says Szasz, there is nothing for psychiatrists to do; without disease there can be no treatment. At this point, I disagree. Even if no mental diseases exist, the rituals practised by psychiatrists are important and valuable. My complaint is that my psychiatric colleagues, convinced that their ministrations are rational and scientific, conclude that our patients are biologically or psychologically inferior to the rest of us.

In *fin-de-siècle* Vienna, Karl Kraus dissected the rampant hypocrisy and illogic he saw around him. He noted that, like biologists, psychoanalysts think they are discovering final truths about humans. They forget, he reminded his readers, that psychoanalysis is nothing more than a series of useful metaphors that expand our view of human behaviour. In noting this, Kraus commented in his journal *Die Fackel* that "Psychoanalysis is the disease of which it claims to be the cure."

Robert Koch, a German physician, Nobel laureate in 1905, changed forever how disease was to be understood. His contributions made impossible the last lingering beliefs in the humoral conceptions of disease, still present in the last half of the nineteenth century. The turning point was when, in 1882, he identified the tuberculosis bacillus. Eight years later, Koch pushed the medical profession further. By announcing the necessary criteria — now known as "Koch's Postulates" — for deciding that a disease has an infectious origin, he committed the profession to diagnosing specific diseases only if scientific standards are met.

As he wrote:

+ The bacteria must be present in every case of the disease.
+ The bacteria must be isolated from the host with the disease and grown in pure culture.
+ The specific disease must be reproduced when a pure culture of the bacteria is inoculated into a healthy, susceptible host.
+ The bacteria must be recoverable from the experimentally infected host.

These postulates forbid us to say a disease has been discovered based only on what our patients tell us. If a patient makes a complaint, we aren't to be sure; there may or may not be a disease. Without sure knowledge of a disease process, good medical practice demands that we make a series of comforting gestures, part and parcel of a doctor's

role as a humane cultural figure. We might also do certain investigations: X-rays, blood tests, ultrasound. Even if there are no abnormal
findings, we suggest symptomatic treatments: Tylenol for headache or
Valium for nervousness. But no doctor confuses this with definitive
treatment of a disease. If, however, a disease is discovered, biologically
effective treatments, if available, can be given. Despite my medical specialty's claims, psychiatrists have never demonstrated a single bona
fide disease. *Because of the influence of suggestion, statements by a patient
that he feels unwell never count as proof that a disease is present.*

Analogously, a doctor never says a treatment works unless there is
objective evidence: the body temperature becomes normal; wounds
heal; sputum changes from yellow to white; X-ray abnormalities disappear; bacteria are eliminated from the bloodstream. Psychiatry has
never demonstrated that its treatments have cured a disease. *Because of
the influence of suggestion, statements by a patient that he feels better never
count as proof that a disease is being defeated.*

The best example I can think of is when a patient who's had a heart
attack says he's better. His doctor will certainly take that statement into
account, but won't place much weight on it. He establishes recovery on
physical grounds, changes in the physical examination, EEG, blood
count, and X-rays. In isolation, a statement of recovery or improvement doesn't count.

Strangely, despite what psychiatrists say, they are perfectly aware of
this. How do I know this? It's not because of what they say, because
they themselves are fuzzy on this topic. The proof of the pudding is
that – please note this point carefully – *psychiatrists do not do physical
examinations on their patients.* I, for example, haven't carried out a physical examination for thirty-five years. To boot, a psychiatrist can
practise for decades without doing medical tests: X-rays, blood examinations, ultrasound, MRIs. This is especially true of those in private
practice, where the front-line work is done.

Psychiatric researchers try hard to medicalize things and to
devise tests. But there are no tests, so instead, researchers administer questionnaires. But a questionnaire only taps into what a patient
tells us — his statements, in other words — and Koch's postulates

disabused us years ago of relying on the statements patients make. These questionnaires aren't sophisticated. Two of most popular are the Hamilton Rating Scale for Depression and the Beck Depression Inventory, both of which I've mentioned in Chapter 3. The questions asked are simple, their simplicity disguised by being framed in scientific-sounding language. If a person is asked, "Are you depressed?" and he answers, "Yes," then, eureka, the patient has a disease called depression. Questions about suicide, feelings of inferiority, changes in sleep and appetite, are just variants on the "Are you depressed?" question.

❖ ❖ ❖

Koch's discovery and his demand for specific diagnostic criteria changed medical thinking forever, especially by marginalizing the rituals of medical practice, the symbolic treatments we mortals crave. Non-psychiatric doctors take Koch's postulates seriously, but ordinary citizens are only half-convinced. Patients demand supportive words and gestures because they need them, although many psychiatrists don't fully understand how to provide them. Koch's postulates are rationalistic, and ignore the importance of Cleopatra's voluptuousness, her swoons and vapours, the importance of poetry and symbols. Instead, specific diseases are to be identified, and magic bullets designed. If there is a disease, a doctor can focus on pathology. Harmony, balance, and refreshment, the things needed by many people who come to our offices, have become side issues, often forgotten.

General imbalance is a vanishing idea in medical circles, most tragically in psychiatry — and were humans understandable through logic alone, so it should be. But since we need many different metaphors to grasp human life, logic alone will never do the trick. "Imbalance" is a valuable metaphor, now discarded by doctors because it doesn't refer to any known physiological state. It's been replaced by specific disease targets, a triumph of rational progress that I have to admit has led us into an era of repeated medical triumphs. But it leaves out the heartache that brings many patients to the doctor's office.

And for a psychiatrist, it's worse, because psychiatry is *never* about biological life; the lives psychiatrists study can't flourish on dry intellectual fodder. We humans can't get away from poetry and metaphor, gestures and flourishes. Spices, sausages, and sauces are necessary for any life worth living.

The specific-cause approach carves disease states at the joints; aided by science, we can pin down real, anatomically and physiologically abnormal disease states. But things like post-traumatic states, fatigue syndromes, and fibromyalgia won't let themselves be carved at the joints; no inner pathological states can be identified. And, despite the explosive growth of psychiatric diagnoses, no inner pathological states have been found in anxiety states, depression, and full-blown madness, either. No carving at the joints is feasible. Psychiatric disorders just won't fit into the modern medical system. Why not? Because psychiatric patients have humoral disorders, the poetic diagnoses that tell us important truths about human life.

What do psychiatric doctors do about this dilemma? All too often, having no prospect of following Plato's advice that, like a good butcher, we psychiatrists should carve nature at the joints, they invent lists of criteria that correspond with no known disease state: they try to carve at the feathers. It's panic. Diagnoses that sound real *must* be invented.

If there is no known disease state for a psychiatrist to discover, what on earth are we doing? Why do we call those who visit us patients? And if there's no disease, how could there be a treatment? The answer is that our patients are not in a diseased state but in states of misery, tragedy, madness, and inexplicable anxiety, something that strikes close to home when we note our own foibles. Those who visit us are like anyone else, except that their common unhappiness has got fiercely out of hand.

✢ ✢ ✢

Medical practice is powerfully ritualized: the stethoscope around the neck, the white coat, and our office paraphernalia are props that underline that events in our offices have a special character. As often as not, an ordinary sofa would serve just as well as our traditional examining tables, but ritual props matter as much as our practices. There are powerful reasons why medicine is ritualized, the primary one being our insistence that the doctor–patient relationship is professional. This doesn't mean there is no friendliness; it does mean that the relationship is not a friendship. I wouldn't let a friend in on my dirty secrets, nor would I let him inspect my rear end; my own doctor gets to hear and see all.

Psychiatric doctors like me are particularly adherent to professional practice, and our rituals are always in the foreground. The professional style of psychiatrists ought to be as pure as human effort can make it. So pure that I, for example, neither make small talk, respond to questions, nor answer my phone; I speak only to think out loud about what my patient is saying and doing. My professional relationships are human — only humans participate in professional relationships — but to the uninitiated, my extreme version of professionalism could look *inhuman*. It may also look inhuman to the fearful and those of ill-will.

Why, you may ask, are you so fussy? The answer is that patients don't come to see me in order to air a few dirty secrets or to let their rear ends be inspected; they are unravelling and displaying their souls. No patient visits a psychiatrist lightly. Those who talk disparagingly about the "worried well" and nervous suburban housewives are, I fear, ignoramuses, because our patient's lives are at stake. "My life is going to pieces," they tell us. They come because the goddess Ruin, Zeus' eldest daughter, has possession of them. Ruin — or more accurately, self-ruin — has got my patients in her clutches.

In the security of my iron rituals, patients know that nothing, including their most disturbing and private secrets, will deflect me from my job. The sanctity of the Mass, the call to prayer, and the psychiatric appointment are carefully designed rituals that signal that all is well. In the case of psychiatry, they signal that all can safely be revealed, especially things — dangerous things — of which a person may not himself be aware.

One patient said of my way of conducting her treatment, "This is the best example of invasive medicine." This woman was right.

Psychiatric and analytic practice are active and intrusive — even violent. Although I'm courteous and contemplative, there's no doubt I've resolved to get deeply into my patients' minds, and then deeper still. It's an assertion of my will, determined not to go along with hardened patterns, no matter how precious they seem to be. If my patient is a decent citizen, I have only one reaction: "Why is it so important for you to be a decent citizen?" If he is a fool or a scoundrel, nothing is different: "Why is it so important for you to be a fool or a scoundrel?"

To subvert deeply and take risks, we need ritual; ceremonies guarantee that, no matter what happens, the culture's pledge that all is well can be relied on. To plumb deeply, assurance is needed that all safety nets are in place. Furthermore, to those who are mad, we are saying, ritually, "There is hope, not all is lost."

✣ ✣ ✣

I recently read a book on suicide, entitled *Night Falls Fast*,[2] written by Kay Redfield Jamison, a well-regarded academic at Johns Hopkins University, a terrific school of which my own son is a graduate. Dr. Jamison has attempted suicide herself, has suffered from depression, and has written many papers and books on these topics.

When I was a student, I was taught that people who suffer from a disorder — blindness, post-traumatic conditions, depression — are ill-suited to work with those similarly afflicted or to study and write about these things. Being afflicted themselves, my teachers said, they are biased, over-involved, and have unwholesome motivations for doing such work, motivations that distort what they do.

This is balderdash, one of those slogan-advisories we humans love to put out. As always, both opinions are true: those who have been depressed may understand better; those who have been depressed may carry a cargo of bias. Despite those teachers, *Night Falls Fast* is splendid, a book every psychiatric student should read, exhaustive, thoroughly researched, scholarly. It's also written in a style that, for a medical academic, is unusually literary. It's a lesson in how to write about current opinion and how to answer exam questions on suicide and depression.

Yes, Jamison's book will help students to write exams, but it's also a pseudoscientific travesty, important because it's a marvel of its type: current psychiatric writing. *The book appals me.* Its ostensible aim is to convince the reader that depression and suicide are diseases, caused by abnormal genes. I'm going to rap Jamison's knuckles as hard as I can, not because she's different from most psychiatrists, but precisely because she's a perfect representative of what's gone sour in my profession. Could it really be true that Kay Jamison hasn't noticed that there are epidemics of suicide and that, no matter where suicide is studied, its incidence varies from time to time? The most striking example I know is the Canadian territory of Nunavut,[3] where suicide is seven times as frequent as in the rest of Canada. Obviously, were suicide genetic, its incidence would be unchanging.

Because I'm casting doubt on what we read every day in the media — enthusiastic reports of impending cures for everything under the sun — my point of view, if misunderstood, sounds pessimistic. But there's no choice; it's just not true that psychiatric discoveries are being made, that science is on the verge of a breakthrough, and that hopes for scientific treatments are justified. The only way to refute such claims is to point to treatment practices: all treatments are used for every psychiatric disorder, a shotgun approach that belies any claim that disease-targeting treatments are available. It's a great comfort to think we're on the right track, but misplaced optimism interferes with getting things straight. I suspect we'll not deal well with the enigma of madness until we acknowledge that, so far, we've come up with little more than optimistic slogans.

When I was a young doctor, we spoke honestly: psychiatric disorders are functional. Medical students (as distinct from psychiatrists) still distinguish between functional disorders — in patients in whom no abnormalities have ever been detected — and true organic disorders, in patients who have objectively demonstrable pathology. To say something is functional is dead honest, because it says, simply, that's what some people do and nobody knows why. The word wasn't applied only to psychiatric patients; neurasthenia, somatoform disorder, learning disability, delinquency, chronic fatigue syndrome, fibromyalgia, attention deficit disorder, and many others were also called functional. Because it made clear that we didn't have an answer, it was honest and invited two reasonable responses: first, it drew the concerned interest of doctors, including their benevolent manner and medical rituals; second, it stimulated further thinking.

Alfred Adler, a Viennese psychoanalyst, at one time a close associate of Freud, said of people who suffer psychologically, not that they had a functional disorder, but that they had a "style of life." This sounds like the modern notion of "lifestyle," and yet it's dead on. Those who eat whole, organic, and vegetarian foods have adopted styles of life, as have conventional eaters, those with religious dietary habits, and youngsters with anorexia nervosa.

If I say that schizophrenia and depression are important styles of living a life, I undermine the basic career assumptions of many modern psychiatrists; they are powerfully invested in believing schizophrenia and depression are diseases and *not* ways of living a life. But they are. Devoting oneself to a career that insists psychological suffering is biologically caused is also a way of living a life, one that believes things a certain way. My conclusion? Style of life is everything; it is the thing psychiatrists try to nail down about their patients. Do I have any synonyms? Yes, a whole series of phrases that point to what I have in mind:

- It's just what people do (Wittgenstein).
- Becoming who you are (Nietzsche).
- It's what turns him on.
- Lifestyle.
- One's own, personal placebo cure.
- Doing one's own thing.
- Living out one's destiny.
- Functional disorders.
- Style of life (Adler).
- Personal agency.

A character in John Steinbeck's *Grapes of Wrath*[4] said of people's actions that they were "Just stuff people does." Jamison won't have it. She concludes that these things are not a style of life, because, in her mind, human disquiet must have a cause. This false conclusion springs from her weak understanding of what, in any culture, counts as a disease. To define disease, we need to remember Wittgenstein's commentary on games: there are no clear rules for what counts as a game. The same goes for illness and disease. We all have a rough idea of what we'd call an illness, but, from time to time, we may be talking about a massive tumour in the lung, a fear of heights, obesity, or shoplifting.

My creaky knees and my neighbour's moderately elevated blood pressure were once the ordinary, normal concomitants of aging. Now, both of us are candidates for treatment: I'm told I should have a knee replacement; my middle-aged neighbour — unmedicated, his blood pressure is 140/95 — takes two drugs to lower his blood pressure. People like me who worry that the definition of illness is expanding far too much are also caught up in the wellness fervour. I, for example, don't want to retire to my rocking chair because of arthritic knees. I want a new titanium knee joint.

Our usual assumption is that biological change defines illness, but this just isn't true; illness is a social construct. At twenty, most of us have atherosclerotic changes in our blood vessels, but if it's almost universal, does it count as disease? The answer is that, if the culture so defines it, it's a disease. Public-health measures are therefore applied: McDonald's agrees that the eating habits of youngsters must change; schools pressure children to exercise.

The same goes for madness. The worries of everyday life — anxiety, grief, misery — are illnesses, because that's the way we define them nowadays. Intermittently throughout history, and consistently for a hundred years, overt madness has also enjoyed illness status. This doesn't mean that the miserable and the mad have biological abnormalities; it's now just the way we talk about these people.

✣ ✣ ✣

Stuck in the biology error, Jamison fails to understand this. Like many of my biologically and research-oriented friends, she struggles to sup-

port her argument by saying things along the lines of: "There is suggestive evidence . . ."; "Evidence is converging that . . ."; "It now seems
likely . . ." And so on.

This is bad science and bad philosophy. John Bentley Mays, a
Toronto journalist who writes — very well — about the visual arts, is a
long-time sufferer from depression. While battling it, he plunged into
the psychiatric literature — and was appalled. The greenest cub
reporter, he said, wouldn't be allowed to get away with such silly evi-
dential claims, sly nudges, winks, hints, and implications — no facts
— implying they're onto something of scientific importance. That's
what Kay Jamison does, and she speaks for important elements of my
profession, elements that have, put politely, lost their way. The other
writing trick they exploit is the use of the passive voice and the sub-
junctive case, which is not possible if one is committed to science.

But words like "suggestive," "impression," "likely," "may," and "some"
are good for something: rhetoric, the style of argument at which I'm
adept, and which I myself wield alongside my logical darts. Rhetoric is
honest: it doesn't claim causal proof and doesn't lean on science.
Propaganda is a synonym for rhetoric, the latter being a literary-sounding
euphemism, cleaned up by linking it to ancient philosophy and academia.
There's no harm in rhetorical arguments about determinism and free
will, but when applied to human lives, it dare not pretend it can prove
anything. Good psychiatric rhetoric (my kind, of course) is softer, sprinkled with doubt: "I worry that . . ." and "Could it be that . . . ?"

Dr. Jamison rarely has doubts, nor does she confess to sins.
Because she announces repeatedly that she knows, a priori, that her
patients have illnesses, her style resembles no known scientific attitude. She cannot go beyond saying: "Their pre-illness . . . histories *tend
to be* . . ."; "Bipolar children *are more likely to have* . . ." (my italics).

✛ ✛ ✛

Arguments used by biological psychiatrists count on an assumption:
human behaviour can only be thought about wisely using a causal
model, *pace* Shakespeare, Homer, Chekhov, and Saul Bellow. Here's

Tolstoy getting this point right, commenting in *War and Peace* on the inanity of blind causal assumptions[5]:

> Man's mind cannot grasp the causes of events in their completeness, but the desire to find those causes is implanted in man's soul. And without considering the multiplicity and complexity of the conditions any one of which taken separately may seem to be the cause, he snatches at the first approximation to a cause that seems to him intelligible and says: "This is the cause!" In historical events (where the actions of men are the subject of observation) the first and most primitive approximation to present itself was the will of the gods and, after that, the will of those who stood in the most prominent position — the heroes of history.

Because they've limited themselves by taking on the philosophical doctrine of determinism, my psychiatric colleagues frantically peruse twin studies, suicide statistics, and family histories, always inconclusively, their hopes of finding bad genes never dampened. That a man earns for himself the diagnosis of schizophrenia (it's a moot point whether schizophrenia exists) and his identical twin lives a normal life doesn't faze them. Nor is faith in gene theory weakened when someone diagnosed as schizophrenic recovers, even though it's unlikely a person with a genetic disorder could ever get better. Since those given the diagnosis schizophrenia have fewer children than the rest of us, were it a genetic disorder it would have disappeared long ago. Genes with a low reproductive rate have very short careers.

Because we're in the middle of it, we don't notice we're inching towards renewing a nineteenth-century wave of classification projects, trying to divide people up: Ernst Kretchmer's body types; Cesare Lombroso's codification of physical characteristics of criminality; Alphonse Bertillon's anthropometrics.

Those who believe in extrasensory perception have lists of examples and findings just as long as those of biological psychiatrists, but since believers in extrasensory perception have no scientific credentials, their claims are sneeringly labelled "superstition." This is the accusation made about those whose superstitions differ from our own. I scorn superstition, but I shouldn't be so automatic and sweeping; I should scorn only if the carrier of the superstition is dogmatic and propagandistic.

Like science-obsessed psychiatrists, believers in extrasensory perception know a good thing when they see it. They realize the official good guys are cornering the market on the word "science," and do their best to convince us that they, too, are in the science camp. But of course, when psychiatrists use the word, it's a toss-up whether it applies to real science or to a superstition. Strangely, people who think science's place in psychiatry is limited — people like me — are the most rigorous in their scientific thinking; those who proclaim the importance of science in psychiatry are poor scientists.

The superstitions of psychiatrists are made possible by their imaginary alliance with science. What they forget is that science is not about knowing things; true scientists, like Socrates, are aware that they have no final knowledge about anything, that their hypotheses, when useful, survive. But their value is that they yield practical results, not that they are the truth. I try my best to stay allied with the latter. I'm in the same boat as my scientifically aligned colleagues: I'm bad at doubting my own convictions. Despite my claim that psychiatry has little to do with science, I make this claim on scientific grounds: I'm asking for replicable evidence.

When psychiatrists invoke the word science, it's nearly always a superstitious allegiance they're talking about. It's a hard error to undo. And of course, the word "science" is the goose that lays the golden egg — by opening the coffers of granting agencies.

Being a good rhetorician, Kay Jamison, like me, knows how to use sensational examples to strengthen her case. She doesn't mention dragon blood and Chinese characters written on water, but she gives us a similarly exotic example from Robert Burton's famous book, *The Anatomy of Melancholy*. Good-naturedly, she lets us see seventeenth-century folly:

Marigold is "much approved against melancholy," wrote
Robert Burton in 1621; so too are dandelion, ash, willow,
tamarisk, roses, violets, sweet apples, wine, tobacco, syrup
of poppy, featherfew, and sassafras. A ring made of the hoof
of an ass's right forefoot is "not altogether to be rejected,"
and "St. John's wort, gathered on a Friday in the hour of
Jupiter . . . mightily helps."

But Jamison doesn't let us see twenty-first-century folly, reflexive
prescribing of antidepressants at any sign of unhappiness, even
though the placebo effect obscures any chance we have of knowing
how helpful these drugs are. Nor does she let us see that her scientific
evidence is as flawed as Robert Burton's. Because she uses a modern
language, that of science, Jamison's strategies don't sound strange in
our ears; because he uses seventeenth-century herbalist language,
Burton's strategies sound preposterous. If academics claim they are
making scientific arguments, they are rarely accused of superstition
because grant-approving committees are bewitched by the magic of
words. I pray that mutual back-scratching is only rarely at play.

The anxious insistence that, sooner or later, we will discover human
behaviour to be the result of straightforward causes is illustrated by the
obsessively repeated nature/nurture question: Is human behaviour
caused by inheritance or is it caused by the environment? Because the
question *presumes* causality, it's close kin of the question "Have you
stopped beating your wife?" Shakespeare, perhaps the first to use the
terms nature and nurture in opposition, had animal or biological causality in mind when he had Prospero describe Caliban as less than human:
"A devil, a born devil, on whose nature / Nurture can never stick."

The nature/nurture question is doomed to remain unanswered,
because of the innocence of its underlying assumptions, close cousin
to the Cartesian mind/body folly: I am a physical body, you see, and
somewhere inside it lives a mind, a psyche, a ghost; or conversely, I am
this mind/spirit-thing, thank God, and happen to possess a conven-
ient body, along with its ingenious chemistry and physiology. The
biologists are still caught in the former trap, focusing on the body, my

psychoanalytic colleagues in the latter. Because someone might misunderstand and not realize I'm using a metaphor, I'm taking philosophical risks when, like the latter group, I use words like "soul."

Fortunately, mind–body dualism is such a bad theory that few scientists take it seriously, therefore I feel free to use terms like mind and body metaphorically. I can easily say someone is thinking about sex, but metaphors can substitute one for another, so I can also say his testosterone is acting up. Using thinking and hormones metaphorically frees me to use other interesting metaphors: he has a dirty mind; he is an animal; he is a romantic; he is a fool; he a slave to his body; he is waking up to life. When discussing human actions, a scientist who takes the words mind and body literally is in trouble twice over. First, he is philosophically and scientifically naive, and, second, he's limited to the single metaphor he's let himself take literally, cramped into a stereotype.

Explaining human events isn't done by finding causes, but by noticing interrelationships. In the realm of behaviour, "causes" turn out to be at best partial, certainly pseudo-scientific, and simple-mindedly two-dimensional. People and societies are not made up of linear series of events, but of highly complex and interconnected systems.

The clincher is that, when we listen to and study our patients, what counts isn't what they tell us happened, but what they *think* happened. In his memoir, *Speak, Memory*, Vladimir Nabokov shows that he agrees with me.

> Neither in environment nor in heredity can I find the exact instrument that fashioned me, the anonymous roller that pressed upon my life a certain intricate watermark whose unique design becomes visible when the lamp of art is made to shine through life's foolscap.

Nikolai Illarionovich Kozlov, Nabokov's great-grandfather, was the first president of the Russian Imperial Academy of Medicine, and the author of a paper called "On the Coarctation of the Jugular Foramen in the Insane." The paper had the answer, a causal answer, to why the insane are insane. Like the new psychiatric ideas that constantly spring up, the idea of coarctation of the jugular foramen was never heard of again.

Thousands of such papers are written, and thousands more will be written; doctors are frantic to find causes for madness, even though the madness of the madman is human, albeit strange and unsettling to those who have to live with him. Not only that, causality is treated as a fact of nature, and its enthusiasts forget that causality is a human construction, a helpful theory, valuable for certain purposes. It's a good illustration of how we find what we look for. Causality makes comprehensible a particular category of things, but it's not a truth about why *A* follows *B*; it's simply a way of putting (some) things together.

Despite Nikolai Illarionovich's confident claim, the great-grandson knew better. Something, his ancestor said, gets pinched as it passes through an undersized jugular foramen (an opening located on the bottom of the skull), a finding that no one else has been able to demonstrate; he was wrong. It's easy to measure a foramen and establish whether or not it's coarcted (too small), and yet Nikolai Illarionovich had made a mistake. It's a thousand times harder to detect subtle chemical and anatomical changes in brain structures, yet researchers keep finding them — in new discoveries that are never again heard about. But those who claim causality is the be-all and end-all of understanding human behaviour will never give up. Nor will I.

Many people think the only other possibility would be free will, to say people *choose* to act as they do. Depression, madness, and every foolishness would then be simple choices. Because it's another reductionistic trap, this line of thought earns just as bad a grade. Wiser to stick with Wittgenstein, whose advice was to only say, "That's what people do." For example, I can tell you that people:

+ Invent slogans and aphorisms.
+ Get stoned.
+ Go to concerts.
+ Believe in God.
+ Get married.
+ Visit psychotherapists.

- ✦ Make jokes.
- ✦ Argue with, or submit to, their teachers.
- ✦ Act psychotic.
- ✦ Have eating rituals.
- ✦ Worry about their bowels.
- ✦ Create art.
- ✦ Make unexpected sexual choices.
- ✦ Suffer anxiety, phobias, testiness.
- ✦ Fight wars.
- ✦ Are charmed by children.
- ✦ Do scientific research.
- ✦ Write cranky books.
- ✦ Tell stories.

I'm alluding above to Wittgenstein's idea of family resemblances. Not everyone does all these things, but we recognize these actions as having a family resemblance to one another: all are things people do, the cautious dogma of saying only that something is functional. Wittgenstein raises this point in the context of understanding whether we can know someone else's mind. His answer is that, if we think carefully, we realize that we don't "know" the mind of the other person; we have specific ideas, emotions, and actions in response to certain behaviours that we see. When a friend falls, cries out, and shakes his hand and wrist, we are acculturated to understand this a certain way and to say, "Oh, you've hurt your wrist." In other words, we assume we know something about his mind: that he is in pain.

But it's always only an assumption. We've adopted our culture's style of reacting to a fall, a cry, and a shaking of the hand and wrist. We can't know, for example, that someone is thinking, but if he furrows his brow and blinks his eyelids rapidly, we *assume* he is thinking.

Usually it's necessary to observe closely, to note subtleties. I don't just note that my friend Edward got married yesterday, I also see his body language while standing before the priest, his sighs and clenched teeth. If the signs are numerous enough, they lead me to make further statements to myself about what Edward is doing:

- He's dreaming of living happily ever after.
- He's scared stiff.
- He's annoyed that his brother hasn't come to the wedding.
- He's imagining God's presence in the church.

I'm still obliged to have good reason for saying what I do, because, rather than being conclusive, body language is only suggestive. My assumptions would be more solidly grounded if Edward had told me about his fairy-tale dreams of marriage, his nervousness, his negligent brother, and his deep religious beliefs, but even that isn't conclusive. I'm stuck with making assumptions based on traditional ways of using the information that's around. The only other thing I can do is to make more observations: white lips; trembling fingers; a starry-eyed look on his face.

Every observation depends on my being acculturated. If I say, "that's a bad joke; he's nuts; what a fine person; you have a gorgeous house," I am reacting according to the style of our culture. I don't "know" it's a gorgeous house; it's just one of our culture's ways of reacting in those circumstances. This isn't philosophical quibbling; it has practical consequences, especially for psychiatrists. If I say of my patient she hates men because she had a bad father, there are abnormal chemicals in her brain, or she has a savage Oedipus complex, I will be strongly influenced to think in certain ways. If, however, I stay as descriptive as possible and say only that her way of being in the world is to hate men, I'm influenced to keep thinking. *I'm being very scientific.*

✠ ✠ ✠

Wittgenstein is at pains to insist these descriptive reactions to the world are rule-bound. There is a sort of rule that says, "When a person falls, cries out, and shakes his arm, you are to recognize this as pain," or, "When someone's lips are pale and his fingers tremble, you are to recognize this as nervousness."

We are also conditioned to a rule that says we are to think that things are caused, a rule handy for closing doors, building bridges, and understanding the mechanics of pressing my belovèd to my heart. My squeezing arms, I think, *cause* her to be firmly pressed against my chest. But if asked why I press her to my breast, I'd be better off if I didn't mention my contracting arm muscles, nor would a reference to hormones do any better: when in love, pressing my belovèd to my heart is just one of the things we humans do. Causality is, you see, useless for understanding love, writing poetry, and studying quantum physics and relativity theory. A rule against causality is not absolute; sometimes it's useful. But it's useless for explaining human behaviour.

Roman Catholic philosophy, unabashedly Aristotelian (courtesy of St. Thomas Aquinas), insists that, if only we'd pay attention, we'd realize there has to be a final cause for the universe we live in. Having seen that the final cause has to exist, we'd realize (eureka!) once and for all that there is a God. Bill McGillivray, a childhood friend who intended to become a priest, made this argument to me, presenting it as proof positive that I ought to give up my wayward doubts. Even then, the argument sounded silly, although it also seemed irrefutable. And so it is if we're caught in the common false belief that causality is universal.

Like us, the ancient Greeks struggled philosophically, and just as badly. Like my biologically enthralled colleagues, they couldn't bring themselves to attribute agency — personal initiative — to themselves. In ancient Greek one couldn't easily say "He walked across the plain." Such an idea had to be expressed as "His joints carried him across the plain." To the early Greeks, human behaviour was caused by destiny or the will of the gods; that a person initiated his own acts was less imaginable than we moderns think. In this respect, they resembled biological psychiatrists, stuck with attributing behaviour to chemicals and synapses, unable to conceive of a *person* conducting his own life. It may be — *may* be — a legitimate way to organize the world, but only for certain practical purposes, and safer when used as poetic wit. For example, Lionel Trilling:

> I've been read by Eliot's poems, and by *Ulysses* and by *Remembrance of Things Past* and by *The Castle* for a good many years now, since early youth. Some of these books at first rejected me; I bored them.

Enslavement by belief — in the case of the Greeks, understanding themselves as dummies of the gods, in our case, blind belief in causal theory — is a dead end. When I was a student there, a famous psychoanalyst from Buenos Aires, Angel Garma, an expert on psychosomatic disorders, was a visiting professor at the Menninger Clinic in Kansas. He told us that peptic ulcers are caused by the patient's fantasy of an internal, biting mother savaging his or her stomach lining. Here's how his error took place. He psychoanalyzed patients with ulcers and was able to reconstruct fantasies of toothy mothers, aggressive ones, a fantasy that is the first cousin of fairy-tale witches who cook and eat children. This fantasy, he concluded, *caused* an ulcer. What nonsense! In principle, such a fantasy can be found in anyone. There's not a scrap of evidence that one thing causes another.

✢ ✢ ✢

No psychology can avoid the problem of agency. For the ancient Greeks, only insignificant acts were done by the person; passionate, creative, and criminal acts were carried out in a state of *átā*, "divine infatuation." The beauty of *átā* is that it suggests neither of the lies we're liable to tell ourselves about behaviour. It's neither judgemental — "he's responsible" — nor does it absolve — "he's sick." Because it suggests that psychiatric patients are our protoplasmic inferiors, the latter explanation, the "infirmity" lie, distresses me. This logic relies on the tired tautology I've already complained about: they're diseased because they have a disease.

In our day-to-day lives we don't use that language, often preferring the moralistic idea of "responsibility." But since psychiatry has become a powerful force in our culture, a force that, on superstitious grounds, claims to be scientific, we've inclined towards the idea of a nonpersonal infirmity.

Homer and the gods knew better; in the opening stanzas of *The Odyssey*, Zeus complains of the mortals who blame the gods for their misery, rarely taking into account their full partnership in dismal events. Today, mortals believe in demons as ardently as ever, although we don't call them demons any more. Dr. Jamison is only one eloquent voice speaking on behalf of modern demonology. There is a technical term for our human tendency to deny our own role in events: "disclaiming of agency." Instead of helping her patients to see their own way of thinking about themselves, she supports those who disclaim agency. "They've got a disease," she tells us — and them.

We do the opposite, too, and, instead of denying that we are the source of our own actions, decide we are responsible for acts of fate, coincidence, or things done by someone else: the guilt-ridden father, sure he did something to make his son gay; the African ten-year-old who insists he has HIV because he sniffed glue and scorns the possibility he got it through *in utero* transmission; the girl who says her parents split up because she behaved badly; my fear that a patient divorced because of my too-enthusiastic efforts; another patient who thinks I'm pale because she criticized me the day before; psychiatrists convinced their patients get better because of them; patients who think they have sabotaged the treatment. The technical term for this is "claiming of agency."

✢✢✢

In her epilogue, Jamison reports an incident that occurred one evening when she and her husband had dinner with a friend. The friend commented on the cruelty towards family and friends of suicidal acts. Jamison reports that she was furious, and kicked her husband under the table, signalling it was time to ask for the bill and leave the restaurant.

Her logic was vehement: suicide is a disease or is caused by a disease; cruelty to friends and family cannot apply. "For heaven's sake," she seems to say, "could one say that someone who dies of cancer is being cruel to friends and family?"

Like the ancient Greeks, she clings to one set of theories — determinism and disease — and blinds herself to the best theory of human behaviour we've got: personal agency.

✛ ✛ ✛

If I arrange to lecture in Calgary six months from now, my colleagues there can confidently predict I'll arrive as planned — not with 100-percent accuracy, but close enough. Predictive power is one of the most important criteria of establishing a theory is good, so what exactly is the theory my Calgary colleagues will use? It's the theory of personal agency; that because I *intend* to be there, they can be sure I'll try to fulfill my intention. I have another prediction: were my colleagues in Calgary to predict my behaviour using biological causality, in other words, by studying my brain, their predictive power would be zero.

Nor could my colleagues help me get to Calgary by trying a different causal tactic: advising me about the proper mechanics of getting out of my house and to the airport. Instructing me about the details of how to contract the proper muscles of my feet, legs, thighs, back, and neck would be futile. Even if they and I had millions of years free to try the experiment, the huge number of motility and balance contractions, fine, coordinated, and ingenious, couldn't be performed upon command. Yet if they treat me as a person, they'll easily succeed. "Get out of your bed you idiot! Put one foot in front of another. Call a cab, and get to the airport."

Before I regale them with arguments like this, my theoretical enemies are baffled that I would put the person at the centre of a theory. My answer is this: "You wouldn't deny that I am a person, would you? Nor would you deny that you yourself are a person. And if persons exist, I guess we can build theories about them. Certainly you are quite ready to build theories using atoms and molecules as a starting point for your theories, and they are things far less tangible than people."

Do my colleagues really think a surgeon would assert that her husband is a collection of tissues? That a physicist would excitedly describe his new girlfriend as a bunch of quarks? That a philosopher's most pressing opinion about his child might be that he is making a truth claim?

On the day biology or brain chemistry predicts human behaviour, we would quickly abandon all talk of hopes, fears, aims, goals, wishes, intentions, will power, guilt, dreams, genius, and hope. Were we successfully understood to be mechanisms, humanity would be shed, including its most vital warehouses: literature, cultural habits.

The more philosophically devastating truth is that all "real" things — people, atoms, cultures — are things in our minds, inventions, constructs, *theories*. The only thing that counts is whether there's any value in using one construct or another. Atoms and molecules are useless for predicting human behaviour; on the other hand, atoms and molecules are wonderful ways of understanding and dealing with disorders of body chemistry or physiology. Psychiatry, despite its loud claims, has never identified any physiological disorders in its patients — and never will. Depression can't be diagnosed by measuring the amount of serotonin in a synaptic cleft; it's diagnosed by talking to the person about his way of life and his personal sense of himself.

※ ※ ※

We think we're rational but we're not. Although Kay Jamison must know the cruelty inherent in every suicidal act, she also doesn't want to know it, especially when her friend's remarks remind her of her own suicide attempts. Her doublethink is explainable only using the theory of personal agency: she doesn't want to know how awful it was that she tried to kill herself. What conclusion can be drawn from noting her flawed thinking? Only that she's a mortal like all the rest of us. Just as self-serving, self-deceiving, just as mad. She doesn't have a disease; if I said she did, I would demean and insult her. *You are biologically tainted*, I'd be saying. Jamison has the same address as I do; she's an inhabitant of the human madhouse.

What about her friend, the man in the restaurant who told Jamison that suicide is an act of cruelty? According to her theories, she shouldn't have angrily left the restaurant because, since brains cause behaviour, misbehaving synapses and chemicals made him do it. She should therefore have forgiven him — if her brain was inclined to do so. I use a different theory. To me it's a moral issue, and, if he knew Jamison had attempted suicide, his insensitivity was improper and he was responsible for it. In other words, he was being a boor.

✢ ✢ ✢

Philosophical stances aren't just hot air. They suggest practical ways of understanding the world, and are judged valuable on various grounds. I like to apply to philosophy the same criteria used to test the value of scientific theories: Are they practical? Is there beauty (like the double-helix theory) in their construction? Do they provoke thought and invite further investigations? Have they predictive power?

Causal theory is Newtonian, and Newtonian physics works very well indeed: we can build bicycles, skyscrapers, or a tower of blocks, and fly men into space. Free will, on the other hand, is handy for moral life: if your boyfriend doesn't show up for a date, you can hold him responsible, as responsible for his misdeed as a traffic violator, a patient who doesn't pay his bill, and the surgeon who leaves his artery forceps in a patient's belly. Indeterminism, fundamentally different from both causal and free-will theories, is neither better nor worse than its co-theories, and makes it possible to think about quantum mechanics. Relativity, a theory neatly suitable for predicting peculiar astronomical events, has an honourable place in the pantheon of theories, as has unconscious motivation, which makes baffling human events comprehensible. You can add to this list superstring theory, chaos theory, theories of God, and a thousand others.

In studying and explaining human behaviour, the most profitable theory is personal agency. The person — me, you, that other guy — is put at the centre of things. No gods make us act as we do, nor is it the brain or destiny. If I've opted to use personal agency as my grounding theory, that decision means we're not just ideas in the mind of God. If I act nuts, it's me doing it; if you act nuts, it's you doing it. When I fight, make love, argue, and bang my head against the wall, my brain and body chemicals run riot, as they do when I try to kill myself, get frantically depressed, or write a telling paragraph in a book. But it's still me fighting, loving, arguing, banging, killing, acting depressed, and writing a paragraph, and restless physiology is part and parcel of what I'm doing. As well, personal agency, like any theory, is liable to abuse and error.

Biological psychiatrists like Kay Redfield Jamison cite findings of abnormal levels of chemicals — serotonin, adrenalin, melatonin, thyroid hormones — in the brains of violent offenders, depressives and pre- and post-suicidal patients, which lead them to think they've nailed down a piece of neuro-physiological causality. They'd best think again: when I debauch myself in a brothel, beat my wife, have a punch-up with my neighbour, or sculpt a *David* better than the one already on display in Florence, the chemicals in my brain do the same excited dance.

The worst possibility is that philosophical theories and social-psychological theories will become racist and projective, ideological, and defensive. Fortunately, good science is immune. Despite their breast-beating, those who flog the psychiatric theory of chemical disorder in the brain are not scientists, and have fallen into a cauldron full of prejudice.

No theories are true; under the right circumstances, many are handy for making the world comprehensible.

✢ ✢ ✢

A profitable psychiatric rule is, Never go beyond saying "It's one of the things people do." This rule keeps us thinking, a bit freer of the disabling theories waiting to pounce on innocent psychiatrists, keen on wrecking their work. The mad pursuit of answers is unseemly for a psychiatrist, not to speak of being diagnostically and therapeutically useless, scientifically and philosophically naive, and, worst of all, judgmental and prejudicial, prejudice being close kin to racism. To say a person is genetically tainted is something never to be said lightly by anyone acquainted with the twentieth century. Cystic fibrosis is certainly a genetic disorder; no psychiatric disorder has been shown to be genetic.

Night Falls Fast makes me shake my head in fascination and horror; when I see her mechanistic approach, my envy of Dr. Jamison's fine writing is no longer a problem. Her book is an attempt to prove depression and suicide are not unhappy ways of life, but are medical diseases, caused by abnormal genes. Jamison doesn't seem to notice she's arguing that psychiatric patients, free citizens, should not make their own decisions but should comply with their doctors' wishes:

[It's] the critical and gnarly problem of non-compliance. An unwillingness to take medications as prescribed or to keep psychotherapy appointments is a pervasive and potentially life-threatening problem.

Psychiatrists in the Soviet Union were also concerned about "non-compliance," and those who didn't believe in dialectical materialism could be diagnosed as psychiatrically ill and hospitalized. I hear "non-compliance" blithely tossed around in the corridors of the Centre for Addiction and Mental Health (CAMH) by my Toronto colleagues. When patients won't permit themselves to be drugged or propagandized by I'm-going-to-change-you types of psychotherapy, they might indeed kill themselves, an awful turn of events, but it never crosses Jamison's mind to think a person may have the right to kill himself, nor does it cross her mind that taking drugs or participating in psychotherapy could increase the likelihood of suicide. It's not socially acceptable to think it's okay for people to kill themselves.

Jamison's way out of this dilemma is to insist that suicide is a disease. The problem is that suicide doesn't fulfill any of the criteria for being a disease, such as Koch's Postulates, for example. Her only evidence is that some people act in a way she doesn't like. According to her way of thinking, I could turn the trick against her: since I don't like her thinking, she's sick. The anti-psychiatry movement — I'm uneasy about it; the members are strident and uninformed — is liable to diagnose her that way, but they're wrong. They and I just disagree with Dr. Jamison.

According to her lights, my psychiatric opinions, because they are unusual, qualify me as a possible victim of psychiatric disease. It's the folly of first-year psychiatric students all over again. Once they've mastered a few diagnostic terms, students adopt a new language with which they can gossip about one another: "What an obsessional David is," they say, or, "Janice is definitely a borderline." I'd prefer it if these residents would stick to saying that David is a fussy prick and that Janice is a ditz. And I wish we all would stick to saying, "You suicidal people upset me terribly."

Because it's well written, literary, and psychiatrically "scientific," *Night Falls Fast* is the best possible example I can think of of psychiatric thinking gone awry. Modern psychiatrists petition the world of science for acceptance, sometimes failing to notice the bruised hearts of those who place themselves in our care. We all avoid suffering in ourselves and in our patients, but psychiatry's institutionalization of avoidance is shocking. Instead of expunging mysteries, attempts to nail down causes only raise a new question: why would theorists fear the wonders of human life?

✢ ✢ ✢

Should I be more tolerant of my colleagues? Should I, like Wittgenstein, be a good functionalist and think, *That's just something else humans do.* It's nothing new, after all. I'm writing about rituals, and if this is the current psychiatric ritual, why complain? Or should I write off errant colleagues? Or should I be amused at human folly? I could also comfort myself by adopting the elitist position: "We can't expect high-level thinking from everyone, after all . . ."

If I ask these questions, I'm doing my job as a psychiatrist and as a scientist: I'm thinking.

PART TWO

THE VITAL PLEASURES

CHAPTER FIVE

DEFEATING GUILT

THERE'S NOTHING LIKE IT: NIBBLE A FINGER-
nail; twist off a scab; squeeze a pimple; strip a hangnail. Extracting or
plucking off foreign bodies does the trick. Nothing heals like a shaman
removing a toxin, be it a worm sucked out of the body, the stone of folly
removed by trepanning the skull, or a demon banished via exorcism.

All cures, self-devised or sought from healers, are versions of
cleansing, tidying up, purifying, or getting things straight. Therefore,
we love ridding ourselves of tags, bumps, blemishes, and flaps. It's
gratifying when the problem is visible and palpable; with a sigh of
relief, we see that, if we're lucky, we might snatch it off. Like the god
Proteus, offensive foreign bodies appear in profusion and in protean
shapes and sizes.

✛ ✛ ✛

In 1964 I was a student, a psychiatric resident at the Menninger Clinic
in Kansas. One of my teachers was George Inge, an African-American,

which was uncommon for a psychiatrist in those days, and exotic to me, a recent arrival from white, Anglo-Saxon Toronto. I was filled with stereotypes — racism, really — and I couldn't imagine that a black American would have uncanny psychological shrewdness. I'd heard he was smart and odd, but didn't believe the rumours; I thought my friends might have misread him.

The big day arrived; it was my turn to present a case to Inge. We were a large group, students and staff from many mental-health disciplines, and I was nervous. The patient, a young, red-haired woman in her mid-twenties, suffered from trichotillomania, a word she knew and gave to me as the diagnosis. I'd not heard of trichotillomania before, but she explained: she had a compulsion to play with her hair, pluck out individual hairs, and sometimes swallow them. She'd come, she said, because the habit had become so bad that she had bald patches.

Inge didn't like my smug conclusion that, having hit on a diagnostic word, I'd aced the case, and consequently hadn't pursued her inner world diligently. I'd passively assumed that having a magic diagnostic word, my psychological search was done. To Inge, trichotillomania wasn't the diagnosis; her dynamic inner world was what mattered. I watched and learned as he interviewed the patient.

First, he got exact details about her habit: What hand did she use? Around which finger did she twirl the hair? In which direction did she twist? How long did she do it? How did she decide it was time to pluck out a hair? How many did she pluck out? Was the urge to fiddle satisfied after she'd plucked it/them out? At what time of day did she twirl and pluck? With family? Friends? Her boyfriend? Before or after sex? What did it feel like?

Then, again in detail, he reviewed the historical events from the patient's life, which I'd reported to the group when I'd presented the case. His interview was exhaustive, a wide-ranging scrutiny of her mind, a vote of confidence in her ability to rethink things deeply and thoroughly. I was inspired by the zigzag of connections he constructed between the hair-plucking acts and the historical events in the young woman's life and, more important, connections with things she did with him in the interview. Instead of her trichotillomania being blind folly, it became a symbolic performance that the patient — and the audience — began to understand.

I don't know what happened to the young woman, but I know her trichotillomania was only a way into her inner life. Once referred to a psychiatrist and started on her own treatment, she'd have talked about love, sex, and death, and about family, lovers, enemies, and teachers — and, *of course*, of hopes and fears, of cowardice and courage. Would her trichotillomania have been cured? No one knows, and it probably doesn't matter much. Persistent habit, nagging idiocy, human folly, the weirdness of our species — we all have our nuttiness. I feel badly about unhappiness, but fiddling with one's head only astonishes me.

⚜ ⚜ ⚜

I want to illustrate trichotillomania more deeply by bringing forward a substitute case, the analysis of which illustrates the dynamic uniqueness of trichotillomania and of every other human act. I, it turns out, am the case of trichotillomania in question.

I first noticed it while I was on vacation in 1980. Reading a novel, I was irritated by a problem on the crown of my head. I rubbed the spot with a finger, barely aware of what I was doing. Suddenly, annoyed, I realized I was picking, and when I noticed my hand repeatedly feeling my scalp, I became angry and frustrated. *Cut it out, you fool*, I thought. *If you leave it alone, the thing will heal.*

I hadn't noticed, but it's possible there'd been previous incidents of this fiddling. But that day I paid attention. *Clearly*, I thought, *I've developed a pick-at-my-head craziness*. If I'd done this before, it must have seemed natural, an itch or prickle. Like all ceremonial behaviour, its superstitious and symbolic intent was buried under rationalizations: *I've got a problem on my head*. Once I became aware there was no real problem, I developed a new solution, a self-insult: *I've got a mental problem*. But today I know better. It was a form of human folly that is well known: crazed tearing of the flesh.

My searching finger found the pesky patch. Was it a scab, or perhaps a flake? Maybe a hair, possibly growing the wrong way? Surely the hair was particularly stiff, bristly, black, tough like a whisker? Perhaps a broken shaft? Central was the idea that something improper was going on, alien, abnormal, and unsettling. It demanded investigation and figuring out. And in a way, rather than me pursuing the problem, it seemed that my finger, intent on investigation and correction, had a mind of its own.

The tip of my finger caught the end of the hair. Although it was tiny, I could jiggle it and, ever so slightly, move it. I tested it again and again, tenderly, caressingly. Next, an experiment: could I grasp it? It would be a delicate operation because the thing was tiny, my fingers clumsy. *Perhaps*, I thought, *if I could be precise, the nails of my index finger and thumb could catch hold.*

But the moment of extraction was deferred; my fingertip demanded that the demonic object be caught on its broken end and tested again. *Can I wiggle it?* I thought.

A humiliating thought: *This is delicious; I love doing this.* The wiggling of my demon was erotic. It didn't feel like sex, but . . .

Simultaneously, ashamed again, I feared I would create the thing I feared I might already have, a sore or scab. I would be marked on my bald head. Others would see it. I'd be humiliated.

I hated myself. *Don't be an idiot*, I thought. *Just take your hand away and leave it alone. The bloody thing will heal, or the hair will grow long and harmless instead of being a short, inviting stub — or whatever it is.* In other words, I harangued myself to stop trying to cure a malady that didn't exist.

Finally, came the solution, the curative moment, powerful and magical, the climax of the ritual, orgasmically effective. I grasped the alien presence with my nails, and deliciously extracted it. Plucking the hair produced pain, but it didn't feel like pain; it was joy and triumph, double ecstasy: climactic sex and the eradication of sin. Masturbation and its punishment, all in one package.

⁘ ⁘ ⁘

Like every psychiatric disorder, my trichotillomania was a series of symbolic statements, a narrative that established who I was.

First, burdened with guilt and contaminated by sin, I'd symbolically located the problem, had it in my grasp, a satisfying start to
dealing with it. Slyly, as I zeroed in on the nature of my "problem," I
also indulged the very sin I was getting ready to tackle: I was "playing
with myself." Cleverly, like practitioners of auto-sex, I was sexually self-
reliant, corrupting no one, my sin unseen by God, parents, or the
world; trichotillomaniacs do their fiddling in private. Besides, it wasn't
really sex. I was repairing something, a physical lesion or incongruity,
something with which, passively and helplessly, I'd been afflicted.
Since it had "happened" to me, I had nothing to do with it.

Not only that, but I might have been doing something after all, but
it wasn't nasty like sex; it was tidiness, cleaning up messiness on my
head, an obedient tribute to my tidy German mother. I cleaned up by
extracting the sinful hair, the evidence of my crime, and, if the truth be
known, the sin itself. It was the *hair* that was a sinner. Wasn't it the hair
that caused me to fiddle with my head? But, since I was the one touching my head, I was making a mess: defying my mother.

I could continue to free-associate. My work demands that I think
about my own actions, so I get lots of practice speculating this way. It's
also easy to see the mutually contradictoriness of my free associations.
I covered many bases, logical consistency be damned. I'm like the
woman in a story once told by Freud. She'd been accused of putting a
hole in a pot she'd borrowed.

"The hole was in the pot when you loaned it to me," she replied.
"And when I returned it, the pot was intact. Besides, I never borrowed
the pot from you in the first place."

✣ ✣ ✣

Trichotillomania is not a disease, but it's psychiatric just the same.
Such so-called diseases are symbolic statements, cries or announce-
ments through which people proclaim who they want to be, how they
wish to understand themselves, and how they wish others to see them.
You've just read a series of statements that reveal secrets of mine that
will never stop festering.

The symbolic statements made by patients turn out to be requests and demands that don't seek the obvious response: cure. One trichotillomaniac, me, wants to talk about sex, masturbation, tidiness, and messiness as it relates to my mother. It has little to do with curing my head. Depressives, too, make symbolic statements. They want sympathy far less than we naively assume. If, for example, you cheer me when I'm in a bad mood, I'll bark. Too much kindness makes depressives worse. They want a different conversation, one about . . . sex, masturbation, husbands and wives, rivalry, and all the other things humans struggle with.

Symbolic messages are contradictory, and those who give them off — all of us, in other words — are, like me, struggling to come up with psychological compromises. In my case it is a compromise called "head fiddling." What else could we expect from humans, who are, above all else, creatures living in symbolic worlds?

✧ ✧ ✧

My psychiatric opponents will argue that I don't really have trichotillomania, so my arguments don't hold. If they say this, they haven't been paying attention. One of the important characteristics of psychiatric patients is how different each is from all others, every one a novel kaleidoscope of symptoms and behaviour. Patients fit only vaguely into diagnostic categories. The system has invented tricks to cope with this blooming, buzzing confusion. The two tricks I hear about are the notions of spectrum disorders and co-morbidity, important-sounding phrases with good Latin roots.

The term "spectrum disorder" tries to make sense of the psychiatric kaleidoscope by assuming that, in the background of many different clinical presentations, lies a single disorder. Rather than several illnesses, one illness shows itself in many ways. The schizophrenic spectrum, for example, ranges from its extreme form, frank schizophrenia (radical unconventionality, delusions, hallucinations), to its least-extreme form, schizoid behaviour (quietness, shyness, reclusiveness, caution about close relationships).

This trick lets psychiatrists avoid being bewildered by the kaleido-scopic nature of human behaviour. Instead, they can say a particular person falls on a spectrum. It's assumed this statement contains infor-mation that matters. Yet it's obvious that we all fall on a spectrum. Although I don't really qualify for disease status, it's easy to invent a label that would be suitable in a real case history: "trichotillomaniacal spectrum disorder, mild, in remission, characterized by hair fiddling and hair plucking, self-deprecating thoughts, and ruminations about masturbatory and cleanliness conflicts." This formulation, impressively medical-sounding and in accord with how a good diagnosis should be formulated, is pure bafflegab, not because it's wrong, but because it's been forced into a technical straitjacket that spoils the poetic madness of what I was up to when my little madness was upon me.

When I was a boy we often proclaimed, "It's a free country." Therefore, in the name of freedom, I claim membership in that hair-plucking club called trichotillomania, especially because it's a grand diagnostic title, and even though, like most who suffer from it, my affliction was short-lived.

⊹ ⊹ ⊹

Psychiatric patients are so multi-symptomatic it's hard to fit them into a category, even with the help of the spectrum-disorder hoax. Lest any wart or pimple might fall through the cracks, diagnosis aficionados have called up another conjuring trick which helps them preserve their enchantment with labels: co-morbidity. Multi-symptomatic patients can be said to have several disorders at once.

Although it's shabby medical practice, the word "co-morbidity" has solid Latin roots, which gives it a scientific ring, and suggests it's not to be questioned. It's shabby because of a medical maxim that advises us that, when possible, we should explain a patient's symptoms by using one diagnosis. It's the principle of parsimony, apparently unfamiliar to psychiatrists, but well known to other doctors and to scientific theo-rists. It's the Principle of Occam's Razor, which says, in explaining a thing, no more assumptions should be made than are necessary. The notion of co-morbidity doesn't result from the discovery of more than one disease. It's a way of avoiding the complexity of all human life, a complexity that demands patient description of what is actually going on. Reductionistic labelling invites us to stop noticing the details of human intricacy.

When a patient has an infection of the lungs, the principle of parsimony says we are to make one diagnosis: pneumonia. Only a fool would give seven diagnoses and say the patient suffers from the following diseases: fever; productive cough; yellow sputum; weakness; chest pain; blood abnormality (high white-blood-cell count); bacteria in the tissues of the lung. The principle of parsimony contradicts the silly notion of co-morbidity.

✢ ✢ ✢

Apart from some psychoanalysts, few modern psychiatrists attend seriously to the linguistic riches of what our patients say. They don't, of course, tell us about joy, wickedness, and creativity right away; the entry point is suffering, so in our offices, the first words we psychiatrists hear are about misery. Like all people, patients sit in judgement on themselves, subject day and night to their consciences, an always-in-session tribunal that guarantees that misery is universal. That's why, one way or another, all of us sabotage ourselves, tear our flesh, thump our heads, and gamble away our life savings. Therefore, people pick scabs, mutilate their sex organs, cut and scratch their skin.

This is not new. The oldest Judeo-Christian story is about guilt and the primal crime: biting into the fruit of knowledge of good and evil. The result? Misery, guilt, shame, pain. Whether the story is literature, a patient's life, a myth, or the movies, it always begins with a moral issue, a sin or a crime.

Sin and crime propel forward every Harry Potter story, as they propel *Hamlet, Romeo and Juliet,* and *King Lear.* The same is true of comedies: *A Midsummer Night's Dream; The Cat in the Hat; Don Quixote. Anna Karenina* and every installment of *The Sopranos* comply with the rule that human interest focuses on moral dilemmas. Don

Quixote, having freed himself from guilt, fights against wickedness he finds in others; the Don, you see, isn't just noble. Dostoevsky, in *Crime and Punishment,* begins his story with a crime, as does Wagner in the Ring cycle. In painful detail, Dante serves up the second course: every punishment that awaits us.

Our reaction is to shed wickedness, the toxin, the offending hair — whatever symbol of crime works for us. Ingeniously, my trichotillomania cured me, while sneakily letting me carry on with my crimes. The ingenious mixture of indulgence and self-discipline in such a symptom is what has led psychiatrists to call it a compromise formation. Madness, phobias, depression, and manic self-injury accomplish the same end.

Mesmerized by the crucifixion, centrepiece of human conduct for half a world, Christians count on this symbol: Christ's death purges sin. But there's no mistaking that, in the expiatory rituals, sensuality sneaks back in: a glorious church, its music, incense, chanting. The return of the repressed, we call it. To top up that expiation, trichotillomaniacs like me tear our flesh. But the bearer of our guilt doesn't have to be simply an offending hair; in certain cultures, every five years, the king is killed and a new one appointed: punishment is brought against the king, the symbolic bearer of the tribe's sin.

Every triviality forces us to make a moral choice. "Which ice cream should I choose, pistachio almond or pralines and cream?" We're busy deciding which is better, the most elementary of good–bad choices. But trivial or not, it's a moral choice, and reflection makes clear that every act involves such choices.

And every choice affects others. Should I buy a cashmere sweater? If I do, there's less money for my family. It's also a violation of my mother's rules: don't waste money on luxuries. If I become an artist, I'll be selfishly preoccupied by my creativity, a symbolic crime. Instead of hard work, good sense, and industriousness, I choose something tainted with self-indulgence.

A Roman Catholic who eats no meat on Friday may, that night at McDonald's, fret at five minutes before midnight on a Friday night: "Do I sin if I eat a Big Mac before the clock strikes midnight?" Since it's doubtful that God cares, I assume the believer is struggling with greater sins, merely symbolized by breaking his fast a few minutes early. Guilt is pervasive, unspecific, and refers to crimes inevitable in human life. Dietary practices, including the self-thwarting rituals of obesity and anorexia, dietary restrictions during Lent, not eating before sundown during Ramadan, and fasting on Yom Kippur, are off-shoots of unconscious guilt. In a sermon, *De Orat et Jejun*, St. Augustine put it this way:

> Fasting cleanses the soul, raises the mind, subjects one's flesh to the spirit, renders the heart contrite and humble, scatters the clouds of concupiscence, quenches the fire of lust, and kindles the true light of chastity.

Advocates tell us fasting, like enemas and plucking out irritating hairs on the scalp, rids the body of toxins. It is, I was told by a naturopath, "The Master Remedy." Unless you shoot poison up your rectum, there are no toxins in the bowel the body isn't ingeniously designed to eliminate. My gynecology professor, in reference to concern about the hygiene of another cavity, said it well: "The vagina is a self-cleansing organ." The word "toxin" is a code: without knowing it, those who use it in the context of fasting, enemas, and douches are referring to sin.

Fasting strengthens the immune system, they add. This is more code: fasting strengthens not the immune system but the guilt-purging system, the expiation. Although some rage against "useless" fasting, enemas, and douches, others, believing themselves filthy sinners, will cleanse forever. Any purification will do. If religion is the opiate of the people, so is Communism, psychiatry, and science; the sense of evil runs like malaria in the veins.

The internal tribunal, harsh and uncompromising, is so central to human life that it's almost banal to mention it. Yet psychiatrists forget. They avoid seeing conflict by becoming savage reductionists. Everything — *everything* — is reduced to sickness, weakness, and vulnerability. It's become rare for psychiatrists to steer patients towards inner struggle. Although it's a vote of confidence, today's psychiatrists rarely stand by quietly. Even wicked, *hurtful* criminal behaviour has come to be seen as pathology. As often as the courts can manage it, violent crimes are redefined as health aberrations.

Smoking, I hear, is a medical or psychiatric disease. Nonsense, I say. It's just self-destructive idiocy. But don't get me wrong. Despite provocative language, this statement is a description, not a moral judgement. My strong language says only that smokers practise their way of being members of the human race, their version of self-destructiveness and idiocy. Surely, every last one of us practises one or another version of self-ruin and folly?

Therefore, don't be surprised at nose, lip, brow, and ear piercings, and tattoos galore. On the Internet, are genital mutilators. The web site that leapt onto my computer screen informed me that a favourite penile configuration is to surgically divide the member lengthwise. Even if this site were a hoax, my argument wouldn't change. Jokes about self-mutilation still reveal our secrets. Any horrible self-injury that can be imagined can and will be done — even plucking hairs out of the head.

Yes, guilt is in the veins. It flows everywhere. Our ceremonial cures, fine though they are, merely chase guilt to new commemorative temples.

✣ ✣ ✣

Freud wrote a paper called "Criminals Out of a Sense of Guilt," an amazing observation that redeems him from occasional lapses into weak theorizing. Criminal stupidity, he argues, is motivated not only by a wish to get away with a crime, but also by a wish to get caught; by getting caught and punished, guilt is relieved. Dostoevsky's Raskolnikov is an obvious example, but the idea didn't click for me until Freud had spelled it out.

In another paper, "Those Wrecked by Success," Freud describes a pattern that is easy to find in Freud himself. His discoveries, so powerful that Western thinking and language have been changed forever, have led us all to think in Freudian concepts. Having formulated brilliantly, Freud then went on to misunderstand his own work. His imagined mental drives and structures, which he held as the under-pinning of his clinical observations, were a weak attempt to explain human behaviour mechanistically. The human mind, he argued, is made up of drives (libido and aggression plus a life instinct and a death instinct) and structures (ego, id, superego, ego ideal). These ingredi-ents — really parts — make up a machine, and not a sophisticated one, either. The drives are the fuel, the ego is the steering and decision-making mechanism, and the superego is the guide. Sometimes Freud was clear that these were metaphors; at other times he wrote about them as though they were concretely real entities.

Freud's greater sin was hanging on to his belief in "reality." Sometimes he understood that we can never know anything except "psychic representations," that reality is, in other words, known only indirectly. It's the merest of conventions, he said, to suggest madness is objectively real. But often he retreated and went along with conven-tion. Rather than viewing the world as a continuum between one illusion and another, Freud reverted to the idea that the continuum is between reality and illusion; dumplings are fixed reality and art is derivative. Why then does art make me weep and dumplings only fill my stomach?

✢ ✢ ✢

Assuaging guilt is one version of the placebo cure, and if it's not the only one, it's certainly in play every time we help someone to feel better. It doesn't matter if it's trichotillomania, bizarre self-injuries (inserting Coke bottles into the anus, injecting mayonnaise into the thigh muscle), punishing exercise (disguised as the pursuit of health), anorexia-unto-death (anorexia nervosa), eating grass and seeds (the Pritikin Diet that makes us healthy), or becoming a derelict (hated by half of us, and seen as unwell or as social victims by the other half). My writing this book will annoy my colleagues and satisfy the same end: a penalty suffered, guilt assuaged, a crime expiated. All are versions of the grotesque mental gymnastics by which we succeed in our struggle against guilt. Grotesque perhaps, but characteristically human.

One can add many behaviours to the list: wrist-cutting, wearing a hair shirt, flagellation, trepanation, lip-chewing, lying to trick a surgeon into operating, asking for one or both breasts to be amputated (I've had two patients who did this), playing Russian roulette, challenging an armed robber, having unprotected sex, sun-bathing, smoking, overeating and undereating, and a thousand other follies that are easy to discover.

And what is the crime? It's being human; every human act involves a choice that serves one moral or aesthetic demand and violates another. Hence, eternal sin. If I succeed beyond my wildest dreams, my father is proud and happy. But since I've surpassed him, I've committed the parricidal crime. If I fail (another crime), I didn't obey my father's injunction to work hard and succeed. He is hurt and angry, but secretly aware I've obeyed the rule that sons mustn't surpass fathers. The rules are a hodgepodge, contradict one another, and set things up so that life has to include suffering. Suffering is inevitable, a device we use to keep our balance — our moral balance.

Why would God or evolution design us this way? The answer is a book in itself, but briefly the answer is that conflict is the built-in flint that sparks us into ingenuity and success. Contradictory demands and rules — internal ones — make us think. My biologically oriented colleagues hate this line of thought and believe they've got answers that can ignore conflict. If they could do this, they'd turn us into machines.

CHAPTER SIX

CLEANSING AND PURGING

IN 1997, MY MEDICAL-SCHOOL CLASS HAD
one of its five-year reunions, a time for revisiting our medical roots,
and exploring the unsavoury rumour that, of the 150 members of the
class of 1957, 26 became psychiatrists. That's a lot of psychiatrists
from one class, even by today's standards. It in a way defines us
because, as is well known, psychiatrists are all nuts. Although four
decades had passed, my classmates looked the same; to me they
weren't men and women, but youthful pals. To me, none looked like
the aging colleagues into which they should have turned.

At reunions, I'm out to upgrade the reputation of psychiatry, by
exemplifying the psychiatrist as a regular guy: I exude extra heartiness;
there's confidence in my voice; irony and jokes are tossed into every
conversation. We psychiatrists are suspect, you see. My friends are
polite, of course, because we're all having a good time, and are still
good friends. They therefore speak approvingly of how wonderful it is
that psychiatry has got its hands on some *real* treatments. They're
referring to antidepressants, of course, and have no idea that, first,

these "real" treatments are dubious and, second, that I'm hurt because they don't really know what I do.

I know what *they* do; like them, I'm trained in surgery, the care of glands, and the palpation of the liver. Although in their heart of hearts they know about archetypes, disorders of the soul, and the magic of the doctor's words, my colleagues don't know how fundamentally souls and archetypes are my daily bread. Sadly, as soon as the words "antidepressant," "neurotransmitter," and "synaptic cleft" enter the conversation, the soul absents itself, flees the scene, vanishes. Since there are brutal reductionists at large, metaphors are touchy and thin-skinned, scared stiff because they are always in danger of being assaulted, treated as concrete realities.

My classmates aren't being unkind; they have no idea they're telling me my work is suspect. They want to buoy me up with the news they've received that — maybe — I'm now a real doctor.

⊹⊹⊹

As usual, the morning was spent listening to scientific presentations. "Soupy" Campbell, the first to present, talked about pain reduction using suggestion, well worth hearing. The topic concerned the strange suggestibility of human beings, a quality that permits pain reduction in response to words. I'm still amazed — even though it's been known to doctors for millennia — that sounds, which have only symbolic power, can change the physiology and experience of serious pain. There was "Soupy," setting the correct tone.

Then it was Ralph Baumann's turn. He spoke about bowel problems. He was acquainted, Ralph told us, with a non-medical practitioner who did colonic irrigation. We shouldn't become skeptical right away, he added, so we listened carefully. This practitioner had taken note of the adherence of fecal materials to the walls of the bowel, adherences that, in some cases, had become virtually glued on. With remarkable skill, this practitioner could flush these fecal adherences, this dried-up sticky shit, out of the bowel. This apparently cured everything under the sun. To demonstrate his point, Ralph had brought photographs. He passed them around for us to inspect.

Everyone was quiet, and it's unlikely anyone believed in this treatment method. The patients could believe it, but the fathers, especially the psychiatrists, had to know that, although he was unaware of what he was doing, Ralph was teaching symbolic healing.

The photos were enlargements, perhaps 45 by 60 centimetres (18 by 24 inches). At first I was puzzled, because the photographs seemed to be of the large bowel, except black. Ralph explained that these were photos of a toilet bowl, and what we saw was the *contents* of the large bowel, flushed out of the bowel by the irrigation technique. They were photographs of turds — enormous, gleaming, perfectly formed black turds. The graduation class of 1957 looked at the photographs of turds carefully, courteously, and seriously. Nobody smiled or snickered.

But there is no such thing as a perfect cast of the large bowel, eliminated intact. Even a psychiatrist, an out-of-date doctor like me, knows that. These casts outlined the whole U-shaped large bowel, to a length of 1.2 metres (4 feet). Had there been fragments of feces in the toilet bowl, we would still have been skeptical, but what he showed us was preposterous.

Ralph hadn't pushed inner cleanliness to its logical extreme: total detoxification of the intestines. Certain madmen advocate ridding the intestinal tract of bacteria, mucus, and filth, toxins all, otherwise transmitted from the leaky gut to your bloodstream, thereby causing every known disease. Everyone over the age of twenty, said the particular madman I once listened to, should be radically detoxified at least four times a year and, once pure, have the gut repopulated with healthy, benign bacteria. Plenty of purifying herbs are also needed. Except he wasn't a madman: he was a crook.

These demonstrations suited the occasion. It was the class of 1957 in action, weird and different. The redactors and the purifiers and the homogenizers and the correctors and the customizers hadn't got to *our* class! It was 1957 as a way of life and thought.

✛ ✛ ✛

I know better, but like everyone else, I feel things are going well if my bowels take action enthusiastically. I also know the topic has wide humorous appeal. How do I know? Well, in Pedro Almodóvar's film *Talk to Her*, there is a cameo of a psychiatrist's secretary, beautiful and sexy. The patient leaves the reception area and the secretary returns to the phone, on which she is taking a personal call from an unidentified friend. "Yes," says the gorgeous receptionist to her caller with a happy smile, "as I was saying, I just took an elephant-size dump."

This scene is a parody of the *real* story: women are required to be pure, eligible for sexual life only when it has been sanctified by powerful marriage rituals.

Generations of historians, novelists, poets, and mythologizers have described how a goddess has been discovered at her bath: Persephone was watched by Zeus (or was it Hades?), Thomas Mann's Sita of the beautiful hips by Shridaman and Nanda, and the farmer's daughter by Clint Eastwood. There's nothing about a dump; the maiden is clean and fresh. Once, streaming blood and shame, young woman were exiled to a special place for unclean, menstruating women. Now, finished with such nonsense, the goddess is in the woodland pool, ready to be seen by the lover and the god. But he looks only at her face, skin, and breasts; the mysterious groin causes him to avert his eyes.

The girl in the pool is a virgin. She is celibate, and for both men and women celibacy can be the healing choice. To copulate, *mîxos*, is to mingle with the world, contaminate oneself with worldly things. Best, say the fathers of our churches, to be pure. Forget about the groin, its menses and aromas. Many a nervous youth has been cured of sexual anguish by the Catholic Church's command that he become a celibate priest.

Medusa, snaky locks writhing on her head, was an insanely horrible sight; should we have the chance to clutch her hacked-off head, the squirming serpents wiggling between our fingers would revolt us. In horror we would avert our eyes and not notice that, at the moment Perseus hacked off her head, out of the bleeding stump sprang her two children: Pegasus, the winged horse, and Chrysaor, the great warrior. The stump of her neck was a vagina. That's why we forget the key symbolic message taught by Perseus's slaying of Medusa; eyes must be averted from the mysterious groin. Besides, if a man looks at Medusa, he will (note the double meaning) turn to stone.

✢ ✢ ✢

Five years ago, I walked the streets of Istanbul looking for a barber; it's my habit to have a haircut when overseas. The poverty was frightening, and I thought people might come out of the hovels and devour me. I saw no stores, but suddenly came upon a barbershop. I said to the barber, "Bzz, bzz," made motions of a machine clipping my head and whiskers, and held my thumb and forefinger three millimetres (an eighth of an inch) apart, indicating how much I wanted trimmed off. The barber circled his forefinger and thumb in approval; he knew what I wanted.

"Faruk," he said, pointing to himself.

I gestured that I understood. "Hi, Faruk," I said, and pointing to myself said, "Gordon."

I was seated, draped, and a standard haircut was administered. A boy was called to wash my hair, but this wash was different. Not only did he wash my bristly scalp, but my ears and face. Then, he proceeded to an eager washing of my neck, my collar was pulled loose and a sponge plunged down my chest and back. In the meantime, a second assault had begun. Faruk had begun cracking my knuckles, at which I chuckled mildly. But then he worked my wrist, determined to produce more popping and cracking. It hurt — a lot. I was chuckling, but hysteria had set in and my laugh was also a cry of pain. Was I being assaulted?

Out of the corner of my eye, I could see another customer calmly reading his newspaper as he waited; my cries didn't qualify as worthy of his attention. Faruk decided my elbows were also to be heard from, increased his ardour, and twisted more painfully. The boy, probably Faruk's son, had joined the attempt to cripple me; both wrestled my reluctant joints into unnatural angles, aiming to extract the sounds of dislocation and, I assume, fracture. Though he tried, Faruk couldn't get my neck bones to snap. Determined to be agreeable, my shoulders complied and gave off crunches and cracks in hopes the assault was ending.

I, too, sang out my compliance, bellowing and howling with pain and laughter. Faruk and his son ignored my shrieks, earnestly plying the trade that gave fame to the Turkish bath. The waiting customer didn't bat an eye.

I tipped extravagantly. It had been a memorable interlude — that's why I have out-of-country haircuts — and as I walked out of the slum, back to my hotel, I continued to roar with laughter.

They'd hurt me, but I'd learned there is a place in heaven for hurt, thrilling and alive. But they didn't hate me.

✤ ✤ ✤

In 1956 and 1957, on many Saturday mornings, Les Fine and I sweated in the steam room of Oak Leaf Baths. It was not a pale imitation of a Turkish bath like Faruk's barbershop, but a *Jewish* bath — a shvitz. Les was my medical-school roommate, and his father managed the place. It was not in a slum, like the torture chamber I stumbled on in Istanbul, but was in a rundown part of the city.

The men sat on benches, which were set at different heights: higher was hotter, so Les and I sat at the lowest level. Most of the men were middle-aged and naked, many fat, but all chanted, although I couldn't decipher the words. Then, the volume of the chant would increase, apparently a call for heat. Shuffling around the centre of the room was what I assumed was an alien, the big-bellied boss of the steam room, glistening, wearing goggles against the heat and a 1950s-style woman's rubber bathing hat with the earcoverings carefully in place lest his ears be singed off. Despite the buckets of ice-cold water with which he repeatedly doused himself, his testicles swung free.

Our chants became louder and more demanding. Knowing what we wanted — more heat — this creature approached an iron door, which proved to be the gates of hell, or some kind of furnace, and flung into it a pail of water. He ducked lest he be scalded, but we bench-dwellers didn't flinch. As the wave of heat hit us, we wailed. It was not the laughter-shriek of Istanbul, but a heightened chanting, and, just as unmistakably, a cry of pain. Three times, the wave of scalding steam would circle the room and, as it swept across us, we wailed and increased the volume of our chanting.

The begoggled alien determined that we should be scrubbed with his bunch of oak (or was it birch?) branches. Unlike Faruk, he had no interest in limbs and joints; first he attended to skin. But his true interest was crevices and orifices, which he attentively exposed, then displayed and thrashed with such enthusiasm that I was once propelled down one level of benches, arse-first, a smackbottom to remember.

After one steam bath, Les and I stood outside the little restaurant inside the door of the building. Beside it was a small barbershop. Both establishments were filled with men, some swaddled in towels, others clothed, eating, playing cards, and arguing. I was repelled and fascinated: did the man who approached us one day really have fat, greasy lips as I remember? He'd been beside me in the steam room and I'd seen his thick fingers, the yellow calluses on his toes, and his black nose-hairs. I'd never been exposed to the German culture from which I spring, but Les's Jewish culture was conspicuous: bright, loud, and smelly. I envied him.

The man called and spoke loudly. "Hey, you need a haircut? Have a haircut. Yeah, you, you have a haircut. It's paid for. Right there. He knows. You need a haircut. Look in the mirror."

We were nice Jewish boys (I was pretending) doing what Jewish boys are supposed to do: we were becoming doctors. Men bought us food and one fellow, Les's brother-in-law, barely older than us, silently slipped money into Les's pocket. Since when do brothers-in-law give money unsolicited?

Perhaps the most important conclusion to be drawn from the stories of Faruk's barbershop and Oak Leaf Baths is to take note of cultural power: a Turkish haircut and a shvitz keep Turks and Jews in fighting trim. Although I'm neither Turk nor Jew, and because I'm a member of my own complicated culture (medical, psychological, intellectual), these rituals cure me, too. Those in the small corner of Western culture in which I live have a great interest in exotic customs; I'm healed by being an amateur anthropologist.

✣ ✣ ✣

Cleansing in all its varieties is one of the great placebo cures. Even modern attempts to cure depression are based on the archetypal belief in purification: the depressed have horrible chemicals in their brains and antidepressant drugs purge this filth, a philosophy no different from the mouth-sucking cures of the Native Kwakiutl shaman. The modern psychiatric policy is to not respond deeply and thoroughly to those who speak the language of depression. From that, we must avert our eyes. Chemicals are tolerable, as are the bloody worms sucked out through the skin of the abdomen, but the mysteries of despair (as of the groin) cannot be tolerated.

Yet no abnormal chemicals in the brain have ever been demonstrated. It's the same story: Don't look at Medusa, and certainly don't talk to her. As soon as possible, hack off her head. Don't think about depression, slay it. Don't have a conversation with those who avert their eyes, just tell them they are "in denial," that they ought to face the facts and express their feelings. In this (pretty childish) theory, anger is a nasty internal thing to be got rid of — like an elephant-size dump.

Yes, hack off her head with a cruel instrument, a battle-axe. For some, other violent methods are the favourite choice: whips, iron crosses. These prove strangely soothing for those who, when faced with more disturbing truths, such as the deadly truths of love and sex, retreat to sado-masochism. More civilized, the rest of us settle for pinches, slaps, and little bites. Most civil of all is purification by fire, the fires of cultural custom: beaten in Istanbul; seared by live steam in the shvitz.

Similarly, my family's herbal remedy, *Bittschwamm Salbe*, when applied to wounds, stung — and healed. In truth, *Salbe* was a refined horse liniment, a rubefacient, which means it heated and reddened the skin, like a mustard plaster. It's a well-known cultural ritual: purification by fire. That's why, long after gentler antiseptics were available, and even though it stung like the devil, families used tincture of iodine. Although rubbing alcohol stings, we put it on our wounds: it *does* something. Like a mustard plaster, *Bengay*, alcohol, and iodine, *Bittschwamm Salbe* was terrific nursing care, excellent for the soul. And in the operating room, when Sammy Sergeant, the surgeon I worked for in Vancouver, determined I should learn faster, he smacked my hand smartly with his scalpel. He was teaching by fire, the method of choice for medical students and the U.S. Army's Green Berets.

✤ ✤ ✤

When we were students, my classmate Joe Stipec spent a one-year clinical assignment at the Toronto General Hospital. He had a tiny bottle of coloured water with a glass rod attached to the inside of the cap, and tried to duplicate the wart cure made famous by Tom Sawyer. Every day, he made the rounds of the large ward on which he worked, spoke to every patient – there were thirty or more — and asked if they had warts. He told them only that he had a treatment and, twice a day, dabbed every wart with coloured water. The scuttlebutt was that many warts disappeared after a few weeks.

Placebos have real effects: it's well known that warts sometimes shrink and disappear when treated with coloured water. But for a treatment to earn the title of placebo doesn't require objective change; those who only feel better are also considered to be placebo responders. Because results are spotty, and because cures through suggestion don't count, Joe's treatment, then, was only a placebo effect, and it doesn't fall into the category of definitive treatment. In the same way, because it works through suggestion, acupuncturized patients in China who receive no anesthetic during major surgery and have full pain relief can't be said to have had a medical treatment either. Since acupuncture is a popular remedy, darts and hatred will soon fly my way for saying this, proof that belief in placebos is powerful. Acupuncture, like painting warts with water, works, but isn't taken seriously by doctors because it doesn't fit with logical, causal explanation.

Chronic fatigue syndrome, fibromyalgia, recovered memory, attention deficit disorder, and many other new disorders are examples of medical puzzles that also have no logical, causal explanation, but because they've had partial admission into the medical lexicon, some doctors insist they are actual states of disease. Although evidence is lacking, for those who believe in them it's been decided in advance that these conditions spring from material abnormalities, that we need only finalize a few details of what has gone wrong. These disorders are the first cousins of psychiatric diseases and, like them, aspire to full medical acceptance. Were they to achieve pure acceptance, there would be no need for further thought or study; we would "know" they have a material cause.

The impressive medical setting in which Joe Stipec worked, his personal conviction he was a valued member of the medical community, the tendency of patients to trust what they hear, and the inclination of physiology to comply with our beliefs, all contributed to the success of Joe's treatment. Two other communities with effective placebo powers come to mind: family and cultural remedies of long standing — or so-called folk cures; shorter-lived popular fashions like diets and herbal remedies. What counts is the conviction of the patient and the sureness of the tradition that offers the cure.

Folk and popular remedies are benign and inexpensive, and usually endure deservedly. If dangerous or expensive, they tend (but only tend) to get weeded out. Mothers and friends don't see that their salts, salves, and herbs produce only a placebo effect; doctors are human and also don't see that their salts, pills, and talk produce only a placebo effect. Our job as doctors is to study what's going on, so we ought to think again about our ministrations, but often we don't. It never occurs to many psychiatrists that they might rethink their starting assumptions.

"Why worry?" you might ask. "If it works, so what?"

The answer to this question is illustrated by a remark I heard a friend make when her teenage daughter complained, "Why do you worry when I come home late?"

My friend's answer? "It's my *job* to worry about you."

I agree. It's the doctor's *job* to worry about what he's doing, especially since some of our methods are risky — particularly the powerful drugs we prescribe. That "it works!" isn't enough; even though it works, I'd be unlikely to recommend a risky procedure like internal mammary artery ligation for angina pectoris. To my taste, the surgical procedure of tying off the mammary artery is definitely too drastic to use as a placebo, even though when used it had a 90-percent success rate. Besides, the cry that psychiatric treatments work doesn't jibe with the rapid increase in patients and hospital admissions. Are there twice as many? Ten times as many? It depends on whose figures we read.

Pedestrian, manual-based psychotherapies would probably do the trick, too, as would a pill, but I'm not sure I'd recommend them either, largely because they violate my sense of what our culture ought to believe in. I'm caught in my Western bias, which, before the wave of biological enthusiasm, emphasized talking about things and pursuing fancy psychotherapies like psychoanalysis. You'll remember Yang Keyuan, who didn't speak of his life concerns in the language of depression as might a Westerner. Instead, true to his culture, he expressed them by worrying there was something wrong with his body, a language answered in kind by Chinese psychiatrists: in China, he'd be far more likely to be diagnosed as having neurasthenia.

When I snipe at some placebo methods, I've got in mind *risky* placebos, and those given credulously. Doctors simply ought to know what they are doing.

Confidence in themselves and their methods leads doctors to bring about first-rate placebo effects. Surgeons, who have the largest stock-pile of real, curative treatments, also have a most dramatic power to heal magically. Boring a hole in a patient's skull and telling the patient that fetal cells have been inserted is a very effective treatment for Parkinsonism — almost as effective as when such cells are actually put in. Electroshock treatments work very well indeed, a fact that can be supported by many papers in psychiatric journals, just as can every other psychiatric treatment. But I say yet again that cures in psychiatry are not based on objective evidence; they are the opinions of the participants — doctors and patients — in the therapeutic spectacle. I suspect improvements from electroshock treatments spring from the drama of having an electric current passed through one's brain.

The anti-psychiatry movement, blinded by their distaste for psychiatry, think I ought to object to electroshock treatment. But I don't. Despite the induction of a real convulsion (not to speak of its bad reputation), it is safe. My point here is that psychiatric treatments, if harmless, are perfectly acceptable. They are the ritualistic methods used by psychiatrists, methods that relieve the suffering of our patients. Since our patients have no bona fide diseases, there will never be bona fide treatments either. Symbolic interventions are all we need.

It's possible, of course, that some brain cells are damaged by electroshock treatments, but an anesthetic may do that, too, as may playing football or jogging — usually without untoward effects. Were I given evidence of worrisome damage, I'd join up with the anti-psychiatrists who complain about electroconvulsive therapy. If there is evidence, I haven't heard the news.

But I worry about powerful drugs, and were psychiatrists to reintroduce leucotomy, bore holes in patients' skulls and cut some of the brain fibers of the frontal lobe, I'd worry a lot. All doctors must have charismatic sureness, but conviction must spring from knowing the placebo treatment is safe.

By mocking Ralph Baumann's colonic-irrigation method I have, in fact, wronged him, because cleansing is one of our culture's vital hygienic rituals. In and of itself colonic irrigation is valueless, but that's beside the point; it's one of countless practices that drive home a powerful cultural message: hygiene matters. I'm an expert on this topic, because my family was devoted to cleanliness — we're German, remember — and we were devoted to natural remedies as well.

But placebo cures are complicated. Part of this one depends on the fact that good boys and girls use the toilet (go poop) when their parents wish it, so colonic irrigation can symbolize forced or voluntary co-operativeness, virtue, in other words. There's nothing like a virtuous glow to make us feel better.

What else? Well, we all know psychoanalysts cure people by discovering their patients' dirty secrets. Once the secret is out, life is transformed. It doesn't matter that this is a Hollywood misunderstanding; people believe this and therefore feel better when they get things "off their chests." So if we rid our bowels of their dirty secrets, we feel better. It's a variant on what Catholics do in church: confess.

CHAPTER SEVEN

FEASTING AND FASTING

I'D ARRIVED IN LANSDOWNE HOUSE IN THE evening. It was June 1974, and I was doing my duty as a psychiatrist, sent to the Sioux Lookout district by the Ontario government. I often go to distant places and know what I'm up to: I'm reassuring myself that people in faraway places are okay, and I'm rarely let down. Wherever I go, people laugh, boys misbehave, girls charm, and everywhere there's a busy, social buzz. But not in the Canadian North. There, something was missing. Whatever it was, it resembled death, but it was social and not biological death. I got depressed.

Lansdowne House (it sank into social chaos a few years later and was abandoned by its three hundred residents) is a two-hour flight from the town of Sioux Lookout, the headquarters of the scattered communities served by the Sioux Lookout Hospital. I'd gone in on a single-engine plane that carried three passengers. Most of the towns had no landing strips, and were so isolated they had only short-wave radio connections to the district headquarters, in bad weather no contact at all.

We'd landed on pontoons and, as we coasted to the dock, many of the residents gathered on the shore. It was a gloriously beautiful lake, and the village was perched on two small islands connected by a tiny footbridge. A white clapboard church snuggled on a corner of the smaller island. As I stepped down, two silent men pressed forward, trying to hand forms to me. Sally Cook, Lansdowne House's resident nurse, there to meet me, shooed the men away and explained. "They want you to help them fill out their welfare applications."

I made small talk with a man on the dock: "Hi," I said. "What a beautiful spot." He didn't answer. But he *really* didn't answer. Even though I chattered, he stayed dead silent. In the face of this austere quietness, my attempts at friendliness echoed peculiarly in my ear. I felt silly; only *my* words hung in the air. *When I'm silent with my patients it must have the same effect,* I thought. *Without feedback from me to smooth things, their words must hang in the air, must be exaggeratedly obvious.*

There were youngsters on the shore. On their faces I saw impetigo, a skin infection I'd seen only in infants, usually caused by bad hygiene. My head was full of stereotypes about Aboriginal people, and the impetigo inflamed my prejudices. *Is their hygiene so bad that even fourteen-year-olds have impetigo?*

✛ ✛ ✛

The next morning, Sally and I started our day's work: "The first person I'd like you to see," she said, "is a fifteen-year-old girl who's had a few seizures. I haven't seen one, but her parents tell me she falls down and bounces up and down for a few minutes. She's sort of semi-conscious for five minutes or so, seems woozy for a while, but then is okay. She doesn't bite her tongue, and she's not incontinent."

As the station nurse, Sally knew everyone in the community. She hadn't seemed worried about the patient, so I stayed quiet and let her continue. "Her name is Debbie Sawanas. I don't know her well, but she seems to be a nice girl. She goes to school regularly and hasn't been sick. Her father is a carpenter, but he hasn't worked since I've been here. Her father was sick one winter from drinking too much — I think he had frozen toes. There was a doctor up here and he sent him to the district hospital. Poor guy lost part of his foot. There are lots of people who drink more than him, but he's the one who got messed up. The parents aren't really worried about Debbie, but we'd better go over."

Like many in the community, the Sawanas family lived in a shack, reinforced with cardboard, bits of plastic sheeting shredded by the wind, and corrugated iron. Mr. Sawanas — he'd probably never been called "Mr." in his life — opened the door. Sally greeted him and said we'd come to see Debbie, but he didn't speak. Silently he opened the door wider so we could come in. Debbie sat at a Formica-covered table, as did her mother. Debbie's sister, a year or two younger, lay on a pile of blankets at the side of the room; she watched like a hawk.

"Can you tell the doctor about Debbie's seizures?" she said to the parents.

Mr. Sawanas mumbled. "It's fixed."

"What do you mean?" asked Sally. I watched silently. The parents didn't seem to want the bother of explaining. Debbie watched, also silent.

"Well, the healer fixed her."

"The healer?" asked Sally. "Which one? Was there a healer in town?"

"The guy from Pickle Lake," said the father.

"Was he on the plane the other day?"

The father grunted that he had been.

Sally turned to me. "There are a few healers around. Medicine men. They sometimes catch a ride on one of the planes. I've seen the guy from Pickle Lake once or twice, but I didn't know he saw people here." She turned to the parents. "What did he say?"

"Uh, he just said she shouldn't eat sturgeon no more. Marie [Debbie's sister] shouldn't eat it neither."

I couldn't believe my ears. Sally's description of the seizures — body movements resembling the sex act — had already made me suspect the seizures were hysterical, and the word "sturgeon," because it meant the medicine man had made the same diagnosis, had interpreted Debbie's symbolic seizures as I had, stunned me. He had given her a symbolic response. The diagnosis had come to me in the form of

a ditty from adolescence, of which I was instantly reminded when I
heard the medicine man's recommendation:

> Caviar comes from the virgin sturgeon.
> The virgin sturgeon's a very fine fish.
> Since very few virgins need much urgin'
> That's why caviar is my dish.

As we walked back to the nursing station, Sally said there hadn't
been sturgeon in that area for many years. It seems that, even if there
are no sturgeon, medicine men and sex-preoccupied adolescents are
wiser than we think — and they're also Freudians.

This is one of the great, time-honoured methods of the healer:
interpretation. It's a method that helps us keep our balance in our culture; by way of a cultured prohibition, the medicine man had told
Debbie he knew what she was talking about, that sexuality isn't as worrisome as she feared, and he had reassuring advice. At the same time
he told her adult men like him were safe: they deal with a young girl's
sexuality verbally and symbolically.

✛ ✛ ✛

Doctors, eager to be scientific technologists — I know, because I'm
one of them — are skeptical and think such interventions gimmicky,
fake medicine practised by scoundrels, and useful only for curing
fools. Scientists fear the power of interpretation, convinced it's black
magic, unaware or not wanting to be aware that interpretation goes to
the heart of human life.

Loyalty to family and country, to traditions of beauty and art, and to
responsible behaviour, are all interpretable human practices, as is the
symbolic role of the healer. In our culture, however, interpretation isn't
supposed to be a medical method; our so-called modern world
acknowledges it only in religious and scholarly traditions, a focus on
The Law and The Word and how they are to be understood. That doctors are vitally involved in morality (The Law) and language (The

Word) is rarely recognized. Even psychoanalysts are viewed sourly —
although held in awe and able to make people nervous. Close friends
are surprised when I remind them my patients lie on a couch and that
my manner is enigmatic and cryptic. Our culture doesn't like to admit
its interest in mysteries.

We all tap into such systems so that we know how to adjust to our
culture, which is regularly fine-tuned as fashions and circumstances
change. But we do this blindly: only when a cultural injunction is alien
to us do we see it clearly. Yet everything we do has symbolic signifi-
cance. We eat and drink ritually, wear clothes to tell the world who we
are, and use slang and current expressions to indicate to ourselves and
others how we are to be categorized. We only notice the ritual nature of
such practices if we are intellectuals: biblical scholars; students of the
Talmud; semioticians; psychoanalytic theorists; English professors.
There are the topics intellectuals run on about. We're healed just as
thoroughly by religion, patriotism, family, and loyalty to groups — academia, fan clubs, gardening societies — as by official healers.

✣ ✣ ✣

The placebo effect, amazingly powerful, is just another example of
passing on symbolic messages. We all have our own taste in symbolic
messages: I liked it that the medicine man hit the nail on the head
about Debbie Sawanas's sexual anxieties, that he both understood and
offered a coded prescription; I would have disapproved had he suggested sacrificing an animal — even though the latter would also have
tapped into her sexual anxieties. If the culture agrees, either action
would have worked.

Debbie Sawanas wasn't crazy or weird; she was skilfully living out a
piece of her culture and knew exactly how to do it. I didn't see her pseu-
doseizures but I'll bet they were like hysterical seizures I've actually
seen: evident caricatures of the sex act. She'd spoken — The Word —
by way of physical movements that gave voice to her doubts — possible
violations of The Law: *I'm sexual but it's not my fault. You can see I've
passed out and, besides, it's a sickness.*

She was, of course, giving many messages, again concerning The Word and The Law: *Do you see I've become an important member of the community, a woman in full bloom? Do you see and celebrate with me this exciting cultural and erotic event? I think this is okay and approved of, but I'm not sure, so I'm interested in your response.* This is not to gainsay a thousand other symbolic messages she'd conveyed. What if she'd sensed sexual risks in her immediate world, or, contrariwise, anxious proscriptions against sexuality?

In his own coded version of The Word and The Law, the medicine man had responded in kind: *Yes, it's sex and it's okay, but be careful.* Psychotherapists who try to work in depth agree with the medicine man and think symbolic talk is the *sine qua non* of our methods. Ours might not be the only possible response but it's what we prefer. All symbolic treatments — all placebo interventions — are a matter of taste. The coded therapeutic message delivered to Debbie Sawanas was in accord with common, worldwide practice: a food prohibition. I don't do it like the medicine man; should I make a prohibition, I'd do it ironically: "It isn't time yet to play with snakes and eat babies."

I visited Lansdowne House a year later. Debbie had had no more seizures.

I'm a psychoanalyst, so this story jibes with my training and experience, if not my ideology. Conflicts over sex are ubiquitous, we say, and I'm sure we're right. But I'm not so sure that, when we say the medicine man cured Debbie Sawanas because he was right about her teenage sexual uneasiness, we've zeroed in on all the components of his cure. I suspect that, like it or not, another ingredient in such cures is the symbolic importance of the healer, be he doctor, shaman, or quack.

Since the healing element is invisible, our science-besotted world discounts the medicine man's ways as primitive or old-fashioned. But his ways are neither old-fashioned nor modern; symbolic healing goes to the heart of the human condition. Any person who ponders what he's doing at any given instant, this instant, for example, will notice he's living out one or another cultural ritual: we live in symbolic worlds. Debbie's hysterical symptoms and their sexually interesting underpinnings were once the main interest of psychiatrists. Freud, for one, built his career, created a research method, and invented a profession by studying hysterics.

✛ ✛ ✛

Donnie Eisen was my accountant for thirty-two years. He taught me record-keeping, did my income tax, gave business advice, and became my friend. Donnie was intensely interested in nutritional healing, the food customs of everyday life. Donnie's life illustrates the silliness of negative attitudes towards superstition — the indispensable, ever-present ones — enriching ceremonies that guide us towards living civilly. Donnie's healthy food habits (very different from mine; I'm keen on cheeseburgers, tomato-and-mayonnaise sandwiches, and diet pop) are familiar and, in Toronto, unlikely to stir up interest.

Although Donnie illustrates the complexity of food interests, the familiarity of his habits makes it hard to zero in on them. Some people said he was a health-food nut. Because they didn't share his interests, they didn't see the ceremonial importance — the magical importance — of his style. We take wearing clothes for granted; such a custom rarely causes us to wonder. A naked man on the bus is a surprise and gets us thinking. *Why in the world is he doing that?* we think. All habits are ceremonies, ordinarily taken for granted; deviations catch our attention.

Once a year, in April, I gathered up my bills, cheques and bank statements, stuffed them in plastic Loblaw's bags, and headed for Donnie Eisen's office. He'd offer tea and, from a paper bag, produce goodies, usually healthy things, full of seeds and made from unexpected grains: organic barley, buckwheat, millet. The actual tax work took little time, but we'd chat, because Donnie, although rational and careful — he was an accountant, after all — wanted to find out about me. In return, he told me his stories.

Between annual tax meetings, Donnie and I would meet during the year, see a film, or eat in a restaurant. Then, too, he'd be intensely interested in the food. The restaurant staff knew him, and he often proceeded straight into the kitchen to discuss the menu, including details of ingredients and spicing. At our table, he would pull out capsules and pills, which he swallowed during the course of the meal.

Donnie loved eating, talking about food, and going to restaurants, but never tried to convince me to change my habits. He was curious (he's *neugierig*, I thought, greedy for novelty) about what I ate, but had no mission to change the world. He was *neugierig* like a psychiatrist, madly probing me about my life, and the restaurant staff about food. And *neugierig* like Alice Munro, who insists that curiosity is the greatest joy in life. But Donnie never preached — I have an acquaintance who bleats endlessly about "fresh food" — nor did he try to persuade me to change my food interests.

Donnie cured me of a prejudice, one of those prejudices hidden inside the pat ideas of psychiatrists, often empty slogans. He cured me of the belief that food faddists — the vitamin-addicted, sodium-phobic, fibre-enthusiastic, and those able to drink only bottled water — are all self-righteous and judgemental. My precious theory went further: if these people eat in an excessively moral way, such as vegetarianism, they may short-change themselves on sin; their hoarded-up stockpile of eating crimes would be depleted. Flaunting their righteous eating and condemning the habits of others, I thought, would be their solution. Except Donnie didn't fit my stereotype; he didn't flaunt his virtue, act self-righteous, or proselytize. He pretty well cured me of prejudice against vegetarians and their cousins; my little theory is now a thought experiment.

⊹ ⊹ ⊹

Two or three years ago, at Lakes Bistro, Donnie showed me the bumps on his arms. I felt them, mostly pea- or rice-sized, apparently covering his whole body. "It's melanoma," he said. His handful of capsules and pills was larger, additional vitamins, minerals and herbs. For a nanosecond, dread passed across his face, but he recovered fast. He was a brave man, so what else could I have expected?

Donnie was receiving standard treatment for his cancer, but he'd also made a trip to New York to see about some special treatments that required him to have coffee enemas. I thought of Ralph Baumann and the enematic cleansing cures about which he'd talked at our reunion a few months before. Donnie intended to gauge the effectiveness of the New York regime, and if he didn't do well, planned to go to Tijuana, where he would have some quack treatment.

Although he was ill, last year he and I went to a film, then to dinner. We walked several blocks into Chinatown, where we shared a few dishes. His choices were Chinese: soup in which swam the limp lettuce that Westerners don't understand, shrimp with their heads intact, and out of which I was supposed to suck "the brains." I shuddered — and sucked. God knows what's really inside a shrimp's head.

Donnie couldn't get out of the booth when it was time to leave; his legs were stuck. "My legs are pretty swollen," he said. I helped him, and finally out of the booth he came. "Here, have a feel," he added. His legs, from hip to toe, were enormously swollen and hard as concrete. He had massive edema. We'd sat for two hours in the theatre, walked several blocks to the restaurant, and having eaten, still had a hefty walk ahead of us. He didn't once complain.

Shortly after, he phoned to say he was in the hospital. When I arrived, he was asleep — a sleeping skeleton with a bony white head and outsized hands, the skin of which was also very white. The backs of his hands had wiry black hairs at which I couldn't stop staring. "Hey Donnie," I called, "*Donnie.*"

Don't be dead, I thought. Slowly, he woke up.

"Oh! Hi! Hi, Gord. Wait a second. Let me sit up."

I had to help him swing his legs over the side of the bed. He kept clearing his throat. *A goddam tumor is pressing on his windpipe or a bronchus*, I thought. Donnie had no time for talk, because there were things to do.

"I think my book is in the drawer." He cleared his throat harder. "I have to phone Tijuana to confirm my appointment."

I could see he'd be dead in a day or two, but he was fighting. I was going to tell him to let his wife make the call, but he sank back on the bed exhausted. "I can't give up hope," he said, and went back to sleep, an exhausted, deadly sleep.

There were chefs, in uniform, at the funeral.

✛ ✛ ✛

The following digression into Greek mythology may seem whimsical, but there are good reasons for turning to the ancients; they are aliens, so their ceremonies stand out. Not only that, but myths and fables don't survive for thousands of years by accident. In myths we see more than superstition: having shed inconsequential elements over the centuries, their important truths predominate. Vital truths are clearer, truths that, among other things, are medical and psychiatric truths. Despite being a skeptic, and a cynic, I do my best to remember that superstitions ought to be of high interest.

An important point about myths is that, although at first glance they are exotic, they actually memorialize orthodoxy: honour, valour, justice, heterosexuality, and virtue. In myths and fairy tales (which, among other things, are cautionary tales) minority ways of life are only warily respected. The stories of Batman and Robin, Achilles and Patroclus, and of Ganymede and Zeus only hint at a homosexual connection. Unabashed celebration or veneration of homosexuality, feminism, or minority rights is rare. For my purposes, it's important to notice that, in myths, madness and neurosis are categories of living to which we must not yield. Myths urge us to live out mainstream customs, encourage boys to play at being pirates, girls to play with dolls.

Science is good at inventing magic bullets, specific antibiotics that kill targeted bacteria, for example, but for understanding human behaviour, science isn't the monolith its disciples believe it to be; it's only one tile in a vast mosaic. Plenitude isn't an unmixed blessing; it puts us at risk of indigestion, overspending, and extra-marital affairs. But for knowing something in the humanities, it can't be beaten.

✛ ✛ ✛

As often as not, superstitions are magical ways of dealing with guilt — universal, pervasive, and eternal. The origins of guilt appear in coded language in the story of Adam and Eve: eating the fruit, the vague sexual implications of this, and the penalties. The primal crime is also knowledge, but sex and knowledge blur; the mystery of sex is essential, and mysteries put pressure on us to unravel them, to get on with the business of "knowing" about them. The Bible makes no bones about this: "He knew her," means he's been in the sack with her. And if I giggle and say to someone, "I know what you've been up to," it's clear I'm talking about hanky-panky.

There is another story to explain the pervasiveness of guilt, one I read about in the tales of ancient Greece, but which didn't impress me — until now. The idea is that guilt springs from eating: if I eat, food disappears; having disappeared, it's been killed; if I've killed, I experience guilt. At first this idea bored me. Then, just the other day, I had a lightning bolt of understanding. Here's how it goes:

The gods of Olympus ate no food; as immortals they needed no nourishment. Only mortals eat, make food disappear, and feel guilty. The gods' interests lay elsewhere: nectar and ambrosia; breathing in smoke from the sacrifices made by mortals. Just as, in church, Catholics and Anglicans regularly eat the body and blood of Christ, every citizen of ancient Greece made regular sacrifices to the gods. Before they ate the sacrificial animal, a burnt offering was made, usually the thighbone, which, as described by Homer in both *The Iliad* and *The Odyssey*, was covered with glistening fat, a double fold, and topped with strips of flesh. A libation of wine was poured, the first red drops tipped in honour of the gods.

But one of the gods blundered. Hades tried his best to persuade Persephone, also an immortal, to stay in the Underworld, ruling on the throne beside him. But Persephone wept and wailed, insisting she be returned to her mother, Demeter, and to the Earth. Because Demeter, cranky over the loss of her daughter, had caused a famine, the other gods pressured Hades to let her go. That nothing grew didn't bother the gods; they were immortal, so didn't need food. But indirectly they were affected, because, without crops, there were no animals to sacrifice, and the gods had no pungent smoke to enjoy.

So Hades gave up his bride. But, as they left the Underworld, Hades distracted Persephone with stories. Casually, he handed her a pomegranate. She ate one seed. This was apocalyptic: like a mortal, a goddess had eaten food. She'd made food disappear — had sacrificed the living fruit — and acquainted the gods with what had never before concerned them: death. The spilled juice of the pomegranate, red like blood, also signalled mortality; the immortal gods had no blood. Like a mortal, Persephone had trifled with death, and from then on the gap between gods and mortals was narrowed.

Persephone's crime, although she ate only the seed of a pomegranate, is symbolic: her offence changed everything. Instead of ambrosia and nectar, she'd consumed the fruit of the earth, akin to consuming the beasts of the earth: guilt had entered the world of the immortals.

Prior to Persephone's crime, the gods had acted as they wished, the only constraint the competing interests of other gods. It's well known that the gods were ruthless in their dealings with mortals, and used them for their pleasure. Rape, abduction, and exploitation were expected. The early Greek heroes were equally ruthless; only after the Trojan War did the heroes develop guilt, that essential ingredient of civilized life. I like to think that's why there *was* a Trojan War, to rid the Earth of old-style, one-dimensional heroes, the ones who knew only pillage and slaughter.

The key to founding a city was sacrifice. "Kill your babies, eat the flesh, drink the blood," said the sages. Only then would the *polis* — the tradition-inspired people — feel guilty enough to behave, or, in other words, act like citizens. Persephone, by committing a great crime, introduced the modern world, the complex world of Odysseus — clearly distinct from the black-and-white world of characters like Sadaam Hussein, George W. Bush, or the Ayatollah Khomeini. Ordinary people, mortals, forever argue whether modern political figures are heroes or monsters, a status they share with the pre–Trojan War world of Jason, Theseus, and Perseus.

Can I connect Persephone to anorexic girls? Could it be that, to these girls, eating is avoided because it makes them into new versions of the god-shattering Persephone? Spilling and tasting the red juice of the living fruit, the pomegranate, thereby making a sacrifice and drinking the blood? Betraying the gods who've never before eaten food, tasted blood, and felt guilt? Do these girls fear that, by becoming adults, they reduce god-like parents to the status of ordinary mortals? When I talk to these girls, I think of sex, fear of womanliness, and the dangers of their own voluptuous potential. But there's more. There is *always* more, and I realize I've become clichéd in my conversations with anorexic girls. If I ever knew it, I've long forgotten that, having learned from Persephone, they've decided to pity their food. And can I connect this to a complaint psychiatrists commonly hear from patients: gagging?

✢ ✢ ✢

Mrs. Clement came through the door of the interviewing room cautiously. Although she knew they would be present, she looked at the students uneasily, then at me, then dropped her eyes and sat down. She was plain, and at first I thought her unkempt hair and clothes were dirty. She hunched herself over, arms close to her sides and legs pressed together, and looked downward. For thirty seconds, I watched this spectacle silently.

"Hi," I said.

"Hi," she muttered in a low voice, without looking up.

Once again, I waited silently, my eyes steady and cool. I've been practising how to do this for thirty-five years. She was distressed, but I was as impersonal — and as resolutely curious — as a surgeon in the presence of pain. I sensed her hunched-over silence was a stance, an easy conclusion for a psychiatrist since to us *everything* is stance. I suddenly realized that she'd already given me a chance to take her aback, amaze the students, and to start moving towards her soul.

"I guess I'll have to encourage you to look at me now. Like your husband, I'll sort of push you around, pushing you to wake up, interact with me. Looks as though we've got some of your ways in front of our eyes already."

Mrs. Clement raised her head. "What do you mean?" she said.

"Maybe you saw what I meant?" I replied. "Actually, I figured it out almost right away. When you sat with your head down, I had the thought, 'For Christ's sake, lady, lift up your head and look at me.' As soon as I thought that, I remembered what you told Dr. Iakovlevna (the student who'd done the preliminary interview) about your husband, that he pushes you, and there I was getting ready to push you around. Sounds like a nasty game you get into, that you and he play together, and that you and I are also supposed to get into."

Mrs. Clement smiled wanly. I could see that she wanted to giggle — *not a terminal case of stubbornness*, I thought — but at that instant was too stubborn to let on she understood. I was still looking at her steadily, coolly, and dispassionately, maybe relentlessly; behind the gaze, my mind flitted. Her momentary smile had emboldened me, and I sensed I could move forward.

"Stubborn, too, I guess."

In keeping with her stubbornness, she reacted slowly, but when she said, "Yes," she once again let slip a small smile. I sensed that, despite shabby cautiousness and grim questioning, a secret flirtation had crept into our talk. We were becoming pals, boy–girl or father–daughter pals, and performers for the watching students.

"Listen," I said. "There's no use beating around the bush. I think we've got an angle on this wretchedness of yours, so let's go after it." Then I added with narrowed eyes and a faint smile, "But you're a stubborn rascal, so you might not like it."

"Okay."

"You know, people who control things a lot — I think that's the phrase you used with Dr. Iakovlevna — get into little messes. Men who are controlling, for example, sometimes can't pee in a public washroom and have to go into a stall. Their habit of controlling everything makes it hard for them to let go in public, I guess. Others have trouble releasing their bowels, having orgasms, or swallowing. In all of those things, it's sort of voluntary up to a certain point — no problem if it's voluntary — but then at the end, you have to let go. Like an orgasm: at the end, the orgasm has a mind of its own and takes over: you have to let it have its way with you. Give up control, in other words."

"I have trouble with some of those things," she answered. "I used to have a lot of orgasms, but now I have trouble, probably because of the anti-depressants I'm on. But the thing I really have trouble with is swallowing. A lot of the time I gag when I go to swallow my food. I can't bear to have anything touch the back of my throat, can't swallow a pill or anything."

A teacher in medical school had told us about globus hystericus ("ball in the throat"), a choking or obstructed sensation in the throat, and difficulty swallowing. Some gag as well, but others don't gag at all. With all of us watching, he asked a patient to open her mouth, then placed a tongue depressor deep into her throat, let go of it, and left it sitting there. The patient passively accepted this and had no need to gag. Hysterical pharyngeal anesthesia, it's called, a medical condition perfectly designed for fellatio.

As I talked to Mrs. Clement about her gagging, I thought of the history of incest she'd told Dr. Iakovlevna about in the preliminary interview. What, I wondered, might her father have done to her mouth and throat when she was a child — or demanded she do to him. But scientific colleagues don't think like me. Here are three excerpts about the problem of gagging from my medical-school notes, the first copied from the *Merck Manual*:

> The exact mechanism that causes this is not known. The sensation may result from frequent swallowing and drying of the throat associated with anxiety or other emotional states.

> Globus is probably a physiological symptom of certain mood states.

> It is not associated with a specific psychiatric disorder or set of stress factors. Certain people may have an inherent predisposition to respond in this way.

None mention the "ball in the throat," the ancient Greek theory that the uterus wanders around the body, and when lodged in the throat is experienced as globus hystericus.

"Do you have trouble eating?" I asked.

Immediately, tears sprang into her eyes. "I used to be anorexic. I couldn't eat anything when I was a teenager. It still happens a bit, but I force myself to eat."

"So you pity your own food?"

"Oh."

Mrs. Clement and I went on: her fear of frivolity, avoidance of dancing, of light-hearted silliness, and of horsing around. In other words, she was always controlled. This was valuable information, but, as I collected detailed examples of this, I had a counterintuitive idea: *I should have ended the interview sooner*, I thought. *She would have been better off had I left her a bit puzzled.* My thoroughness nailed down what was going on, made things clear and understandable, a state in which her wish to control things could flourish. Leaving her baffled might have been a step towards her giving up control, even if only for a moment. "Oh, that's what it's all about," she probably thought when I overdid my clarifications. It would also have been good to keep the students thinking.

"It's time to stop, Mrs. Clement. We'll find someone for you. Dr. Iakovlevna will phone."

It's no surprise my announcement paralyzed her: she felt pushed. "Do you mean we have to stop?"

I remained silent.

"I'm sorry. I forget the other doctor's name. Will she find someone for me?"

I smiled the faintest of smiles.

"Oh," she said. Mrs. Clement collected her bags, shifted them from hand to hand, looked me over, and then at the students, and finally walked to the door. Once she'd opened the door, she had to pause again for an instant, but when she couldn't evoke reassuring remarks from me (the students were dying to ease her passage through the door, but wouldn't have dared), finally, out she went.

✤ ✤ ✤

Why bother with the Greeks? Because they knew something we are reluctant to acknowledge: customs are just as valuable — maybe more valuable — than laws. Customs are well-tested, reliable guides to behaviour; as in the case of O. J. Simpson, laws can be twisted by oratory and propaganda.

Why tell the story of Donnie Eisen? If my aim is to talk about anorexia and food ceremonies, there are plenty of official patients — Mrs. Clement for example — whose case reports I could reproduce. But we're used to anorexics, the obese, and bulimics; the newspapers have made them a commonplace, so their behaviour no longer awakens our suspicions of superstitious underpinnings. More important, doctors have made sure they've got medical labels, so we don't think about the symbolism any more. Astonishment at their weird and magic thinking has been short-circuited. The magic of ordinary eating rituals can stay invisible, but we must be alert to the symbolic behavior of anorexics and notice what they fear: they might eat the pomegranate, homesick goddesses with the power to precipitate the downfall, the *Götterdämmerung*, of the Olympians. If they're solidly positioned in a disease category, we have no need to notice or create new rituals.

✣ ✣ ✣

I may take Canadian lifestyles and food habits for granted, but I'm not used to the eating customs of France. It's July 6, 2003, and I'm having lunch at Sunset Village in Domaine de l'Étoile in Provence. It's a terrific meal, three courses, and because it's Friday, a buffet. On Saturday, my son Karl is getting married in Vence, a few kilometres from here, and I'm aiming to finish this chapter before the wedding. I've counted forty-one people eating lunch on the terrace around the pool. No one has sacrificed a living animal, tipped first drops to the gods, nor has anyone laid a hand on the fifteen to twenty young children who are running around. Apart from offering up my son on the altar of marriage, sacrificing babies seems not to be the fashion here.

But people ate; I watched them eating *moules* — almost everyone had a plate full — then pasta, salad, plenty of mayonnaise, and wine.

The waiters kept bringing more bottles of wine, and everyone smoked, laughed, passed babies around, then tucked into their food, gobbling it enthusiastically. To the dismay of any dermatologist that might have seen it, every last one was heavily tanned. They disregarded their skin recklessly. By tanning, they'd sacrificed the unlined skin they could have had twenty years from now. Despite their lesser enthrallment with eating the right foods and smearing themselves with the right sun block, every last one of them was slim.

I know why: they'd made sacrifices to the gods. Be careful as you read this; it's liable to sound as though I have the answer to the North American obesity epidemic. What I'm saying aims only to stir thinking.

What these French men and women sacrificed, I say, was liberty; in the service of the French cultural gods, all forty-one sat down to eat at the same time, all gave up their prerogative to swim longer, order a pizza, or stay away from all the vulgar smokers. The restaurant would have fed them at any time, and no one demanded that they come and eat. Unlike the Toronto Lawn Tennis Club, at Sunset Village the larger group claims their loyalty. At Toronto Lawn, subgroups, cliques, have priority. There, at a table of four, one person is liable to eat, another to sip a refreshing shandy, the third savour a beer, and the fourth brace himself with coffee.

Although Provence has them, I doubt the standard Frenchman goes to McDonald's. Could it be true that slimness goes with abiding by rules, including rules such as those once followed in Canada: on Sundays families eat dinner together; no one picks up a fork until Mother has picked up hers; people start and stop together; phone calls, television, stereo, and radio are sacrificed. At Sunset Village, club members eat together.

Could it be that anorexic girls with deadly food habits are crying out for the rituals of which they've been robbed? Are dieters and food faddists searching for rituals when they explore new foods? Does straying from the laws of God lead people to invent new practices like fast food, fasting, and faddism? And could it be that, unlike the time-tested Mayan ceremonies I'll describe in Chapter 12, these new rituals haven't yet got the kinks out of them — and maybe never will?

Reinstating family dinners and making anorexic girls join in won't solve anything. What counts is noticing what we're up to, realizing that, like the French here in Domaine de l'Étoile, our eating habits, including those of anorexics, are rituals. We're spilling out symbolic messages, codified speech, but unaware of it. Were psychiatrists to pay attention, might we have better conversations with anorexic patients?

Many Canadians are obese, and our diets are full of fat — and Americans are worse.[1] Could it be that low-calorie foods in supermarkets are useless, fit no cultural ceremony, and make insufficient demands for sacrifice? Then we dishonour the ceremony further by announcing that these foods have great advantages, that it's "easy" to eat fewer calories, that *no sacrifice is necessary.* Our culture has lost a deep piece of knowledge; we humans are obligated to make demands on ourselves, *make sacrifices.* Here is an aphorism of Nietzsche's, my all-time favourite:

> I want to make things *as hard* for myself as they have ever been for anybody: only under this pressure do I have a *clear* enough *conscience* to possess something few men have or have ever had — *wings,* so to speak.

This aphorism is so psychologically important that I know it by heart. Its power is less obvious to the young, but the thought-sacrifice of attending to it pays off. And by the way: the example of the French feasters at Sunset Village — they're finally polishing off the last of their wine and the husbands are going back to work — teaches us that the sacrifice can be joyous.

When we become too logical and self-conscious about how to live, we forget tradition. A catalogue of murder, tyranny, and treachery has always resulted when, historically, it's been decided there is a logical or scientific way to run a country or an empire. Machiavelli, for example, ushered in a diabolical system that worked — and let evil out of the box. A parliamentary government like Canada's works (for now) because it runs on traditions, time-tested and reliable. Eating, too, works best if we do it traditionally; rational schemes that encourage fast food and energy bars miss the point. Traditional eating rituals are designed — albeit invisibly — to keep us safe.

⁜ ⁜ ⁜

Alcoholic drinks are not allowed in hospitals, but with nudges and winks, our medical-school teachers showed us how to sneak around the rules by prescribing the medicinal-sounding vitamin B-complex (in a sherry base). I'm sure the patients loved their little glasses of sherry.

> *Rx*
> *Elixir B-complex* ℥ $\overline{iss}$
> *Sig:* $\overline{ss}$ *hr arc. p.m.*

> Take thou of
> Elixir of B-complex one and a half ounces
> Instruction: half an hour before eating, in the evening

It's the kind of story every doctor should remember. One of the most important instructions we give to patients, nowadays neglected, should be, "Well, you're a bit rundown. You've been through a lot recently, and you should take an ounce and a half of this tonic every night a half hour before dinner. It'll give you an appetite and help get you back on the ball."

Or, "I'll write you out a prescription for caffeine and citric acid. It can't do any harm. I find it's always the best thing."

CHAPTER EIGHT

AFFIRMING WHO WE ARE

LOVE IS THE BEST CURE OF ALL. WOES, anguish, hurts: all fade in its wake. Countless experiences can be enlisted to the same end. In the traditional healing situation, the cultural role of healer is primary. If the culture grants him the prestige and authority to heal, his methods work. Most doctors proudly accept this role. Surprisingly, some doctors shy away from consciously embracing our charismatic influence, especially when they define themselves as technological adepts. We do repair abnormal hearts, eliminate infections, and correct or contain physiological aberrations. But much of the time (many doctors are disappointed about this), we're called on to do magic.

If a grandchild breaks a leg, can't breathe, or has a fit, my adult children know the problem requires medical technology, and they go straight to the hospital; if they phone me for advice, it means they're uncertain. Then, their question is different, and they suspect — not consciously — that the child's complaint is symbolic: "Should we take Alex to the doctor? He's complaining that . . ." Because I'm both a doctor and the grandparent, my role is ambiguous, and I usually don't have to give techno-physiological advice. Recently I was reminded that self-designed symbolism can work just as well as the official cultural ones.

✣ ✣ ✣

One morning, at the corner of Harbord and St. George streets in Toronto, a busy intersection in the middle of the university campus, I'd pulled my bike over to the curb at a red light. Beside me, also riding a bike, was a middle-aged woman. In the centre of the road a young woman had walked against the light and become trapped between the two streams of traffic. She looked quickly to the right and left, then put her hands over her ears and squealed. She also adopted a special posture: back arched daintily, knees slightly bent, head tipped to one side, fingers splayed asymmetrically from the side of her head like the ankle-wings of Mercury. I'll come clean: deftly, prettily, she was sticking out her fanny. This is not just an aesthetic appreciation of the female form. The fact that she was being sexy is central to my argument.

I turned to the cyclist beside me and said, "She thinks if she squeals and sticks out her po-po, she's safe." The woman chuckled in agreement.

This cure was self-created; no doctor prescribed a hormone injection, nor did anyone advise the symbolic reinforcement of her womanliness, yet this young woman's actions gave her comfort and made her feel safe. What did her squeal and special posture accomplish? If one of our myths is the rescue of the maiden in distress, this young woman was ripe for rescue: a girl, young, radiating womanliness, her gender in the final stages of consolidation. Could it be that affirming femininity made her feel safe?

Of course. Proud womanhood has carried the day since Eve's wishes led man straight to the ultimate danger: knowing too much. Knowing what? Everything: the fallibility of God; the truth about love and sex; life outside the coziness of the family.

Less commonly, proud effeminacy carries the day, and, for many lesbians, so does pride in being butch. And those whose proud way of life is resolutely asexual, when endangered, will affirm this with might and main. But the dominant culture celebrates common ways of living: men who flex muscles; women who show off curves.

Men practise the same trick as women, and examples range from sports behaviour to that of the warriors of the Trojan War. I'm not a basketball fan, but I'm told that, in the heat of the game, players denounce and insult their opponents: trash talk. Trojan and Achaean soldiers in *The Iliad* did it, too, threw insults and made exaggerated threats, an exact equivalent of the trash talk of basketball players: "entrails"; "fed to the dogs"; "go down within the house of Hades."

The king of trash talk? Muhammad Ali.

Why do they do this? Well, they're charging up their manliness. They're afraid, of course, afraid of death, defeat, loss of maleness, so they exaggerate life, victory, and masculinity. This is what the young woman did when caught in traffic. In her mind, affirmation, and strengthening of who she was, did the trick.

But don't misunderstand; this is no advocacy of macho falseness or histrionic silliness. Mawkish bravado in either sex is a failure, not achievement. I'm pointing at the joy and sureness of being what we are, in this instance, man or woman. There are examples of grotesque mis-understandings of gender affirmation, such as doctors who think they're curing patients by having sex with them. I've been on psychi-atric ethics committees, and almost every time, the doctor thought his (woman) patient to be vulnerable, and by becoming her lover, he aimed to heal, strengthen, and cure her. Humbert Humbert, scorner of things psychiatric and psychoanalytic, fancied himself Lolita's "therapist."

It's nothing new. In a celebrated case in the village of Möttlingen in nineteenth-century Germany, the Reverend Blumhardt cured Gottliebin Dittus of demons. His exorcism involved epic struggle; like modern analysts, he battled her demons for years. Colossal struggle is an excellent tactic for achieving a ceremonial cure. In those days, of course, pathological forces were called demons rather than what is now in fashion: chemical imbalances, bad maternal introjects, recovered memories, previous lives. Finally, after heroic struggles, Gottliebin Dittus was cured. The passionate, emotionally over-wrought interactions between healer and patient are a story familiar to psychiatrists, and it's no surprise she later became a member of the Reverend Blumhardt's household.

In the era of science, many hope for or dream up evidence of identifiable causes, but there are none. The Reverend Blumhardt, who succumbed to his hysterical patient Gottliebin Dittus — as she succumbed to his overwrought involvement — had no evidence of otherworldly demons, nor do we have evidence, in our case, of chemical or neurophysiological demons, only people madly living out human absurdity.

The story of a Prince Charming who rescues a maiden-in-distress works in reverse, too. Muses transform ordinary men into superb men. Odysseus, no longer young, was an intruder in the land of the Phaeacians. Nausicaä, the white-armed princess, daughter of King Ancinoüs, found Odysseus on the beach, naked and wretched, and in danger from the rulers of that private country. By making his maleness more alive, and by giving Nausicaä the wisdom to see it, the goddess Athena saved Odysseus' life. She transformed an aging, exhausted wanderer into beautiful manhood, rippling with muscles. She crowned him with golden curls and poured splendour over his head and shoulders.

Athena, the goddess with the lovely braids, performed a similar service for Odysseus' son. When Telemachus set off to search for his father, he had to visit the court of Menelaus, the redheaded king of Sparta. Just as she'd transformed Odysseus, Athena transformed the twenty-year-old pup, Telemachus, into glittering manhood, thereby making him a more eloquent spokesman on behalf of his father.

Although bright-eyed Athena gave Odysseus and Telemachus the appearance of physical strength, her ultimate gift to them was wisdom. Odysseus was the wisest of all the Greeks — Athena, goddess of wisdom, was always his mentor — and she counselled Telemachus when his life was in crisis. Only the female has the *mêtis*, the intelligence that preordains action in the silence of the mind. Men and gods know how to rape and slice off testicles, but without *mêtis*, they are only brutes.

Tarzan's Jane, Heidi, Rick's Ilsa in *Casablanca*, Captain von Trapp's Maria in *The Sound of Music* — each story celebrates the culture's preferred prototypes and archetypes, the paradigmatic man and woman, so to speak. It's the same story as the rescuer of the goddess in the emerald pool. Commonly, the wise man knows his limitations, and willingly appropriates wisdom from a woman. On his own, he's just a warrior and a noisemaker.

Had Athena tired of performing the complex miracles she wrought, she could have waited for the discoveries of the Anglo-Saxons a few millennia later:

> If a man be insufficiently virile, boil agrimony in milk; then you will excite it. If a man be overly virile, boil it in Welsh Ale; he is to drink it at night, fasting.

These, respectively, were the Viagra and saltpetre of the Anglo-Saxons in A.D. 1000. The seventeenth century had its own confident cure for impotence and frigidity in men: they should listen to a lively air played on a holly flute or a soft air played on a hellebore flute (or one made of larkspur or iris stems). And if Pallas Athena had waited until the twentieth century, she would have had another choice, this remedy from Vikram Seth's *A Suitable Boy*, a fragment of modern India:

> Does it stand, but not straight enough? . . . Leaning left like the Marxist–Leninist Party? To the right, like the Jan Sangh fascists? Or wobbling mindlessly in the middle, like the Congress Party? Fear not, for it can be straightened! . . . try my ointment, and it will become hard as the government's heart! . . . Capable of turning all men into engine-drivers! . . . The railways and your wife will be proud of you! Apply it twice a day, and she will have to share you with the whole block!

The peddlers and users of placebos live on forever. Here's one from a Toronto subway train:

> Sexual dysfunction affects a high percentage of the human population, denying them the pleasures of a truly satisfying

sex life. However, *modern scientific research* now provides many solutions that enhance male and female sex response and sexual performance. Viagra, perhaps the most dramatic, is only one of many new and proven sex stimulants. Fast multiple female orgasms; strong, long-lasting; male and female sexual response enhancement; hard penis erections; control premature ejaculation; satisfying sexual intercourse —all these are now attainable by all. The promise of pleasure and satisfaction. [my italics]

✛ ✛ ✛

Orgasms are fine and important, but they have to share the limelight. The satisfaction of lovemaking lies, not in orgasms, but in a ceremonial reaffirmation of one's gender preference, usually maleness and femaleness. By her every action, a woman symbolically cries out to her lover that he is powerfully masculine. The whimpers and movements of love inspire him into more fully knowing his maleness. And he, inspirational in his own right, symbolically awakens and makes obvious her womanliness. Fine lovemaking, symbolic theatre of the highest quality, proves and reassures us that gender — and life itself — is intact and worthy. And when it works well, it's wonderful.

Affirming gender isn't the traditional way of thinking about placebo — which is usually seen as a pill, a gesture, or a potion — but it's a healing ceremony of the best kind, called superstition only by those who hate life. It shows off the principles that make placebos work, confirming that we're okay because we're solidly in our culture. Lovemaking is symbolic and ceremonial; that's why it cures us of our woes. The placebo effect goes to the heart of the human condition, taps into our deepest desires, hopes, and fears. If we're all looking for sublime redemption, placebos are an example of it, one of the great human needs.

And what of the sublime do we pursue? Each of us is unique. Some seek God, others aesthetic fulfillment. Intellectual prowess, money, power, adventurous sexuality, tyranny, security, and family values are examples of aims that can be elevated to sublime status, to ideals; any human activity can be sanctified and carry the burden of being the meaning of life. To some, rape and perversion take centre stage. No single satisfaction is enough; all of us have an array of transcendent goals that suit us and *make us who we are.*

It's hard to fathom why some elevate to transcendent status the pursuit of self-injury: criminals, drunks, derelicts, and fools, not to speak of those who repeatedly alienate those they love, lose jobs, and crash cars. Yet we all know that marital squabbling and international stupidity will go on forever. Circumstances count, of course, but, one way or another, all of us pursue unappealing roles. Although history throws up the array of inspirational stories we eventually get to choose from, each person make his or her own decision: not everyone is inspired by gambling or medical placebos, and not everyone is helped by the glory of God.

I'm sorry when doctors mislead people into believing they have diseases when they really need wise talk. I'm irritated to have found these posters (they're not about gender affirmation, but are similar to the silly advertisements I've quoted from Anglo-Saxons and the Toronto subway train) on the bulletin board outside my office, ostensibly aiming to identify poor souls who suffer from disease for which they need treatment. Like the hilarious sexual-enhancement advertisements I've quoted, they aim to convince worried people that they have diseases — but these advertisements are in a hospital. At the bottom of both were multiple little tear sheets — the kind used for renting apartments or hiring housepainters — printed with the phone numbers.

ADOLESCENTS: ARE YOU DEPRESSED?

If you are between 13–18 years of age and suffer from any of the following symptoms:

+ feel sad or blue or down in the dumps
+ having trouble sleeping or getting out of bed
+ experiencing loss of appetite or weight loss
+ feel anxious or tense
+ feel tired or fatigued

You may be eligible to participate in an adolescent depression research study. The study is being conducted by Dr. L. in the Mood and Anxiety Program at the Centre for Addiction and Mental Health. If you would like to know more about the study, please contact . . .

DO YOU HAVE A GAMBLING PROBLEM?
ARE YOU OFTEN ANGRY?
If you are a male aged 18 and over you may be eligible to participate in a study comparing different treatments for problem gambling.
Compensation and transit expenses covered.
For more information, please call: . . .

These bulletins, officially stamped as "Approved for Posting," are examples of the defining concern of modern academic psychiatry: spin. It's a peculiar spin; the "investigators" will have learned it from politicians, business practices, and pharmaceutical houses: sell the public on the idea of a disease. We're not surprised when political parties blatantly spin what they're up to, but university researchers are thought to be — and should be — above this sort of spin.

In the banal foreground of their minds, doctors who do superficial research usually believe in what they're doing, but a lot of current research has little to do with relieving human suffering. The researchers, probably ambitious young doctors or psychologists, are part of a massively flawed research enterprise that spends millions of dollars every year producing worthless studies that advance academic careers. Day in and day out, they wrack their brains for eye-catching projects that, if properly packaged, might get funded. Funding earns academic approval, something akin to getting their names in the paper. It's a psychiatric spectrum disorder: "publicity-derangement syndrome, grant-seeking type."

I love the hilarious advertisements on subway trains that assure me there is hope for wrinkled skin, a droopy appendage, and, of special interest to me, my shining scalp. I'm appalled at academic doctors who, cheaply ambitious (could it be that they are just dumb?), have forgotten their medical duty and joined forces with *Cosmopolitan* magazine and the "Dear Abby" column. I blame drug companies less; it's obvious they are out to make money. Their philanthropic claims are widely understood to be window dressing, but the public listens to doctors and professors.

These people would argue that research has produced important new knowledge, that there is an increased awareness and use of short-term treatments like CBT (cognitive behaviour therapy: persuading people to think differently, usually following a manual), and IPT (interpersonal therapy: concentrating on two or three relationship issues). Were that so, I'd be out of business. The truth is that psychiatrists who want psychotherapy for themselves visit people like me; they also pick and choose the patients they refer to me: professors, actors, and professionals. I wonder why fancy folk all happen to need a psychiatrist like me, and ordinary folk happen to need CBT and IPT? Here's the scoop: CBT and IPT are easy procedures to research and that's where the money is — the professional-advancement money.

Methods like CBT and IPT are a simple variant on behaviourism. The idea is that approved behaviour is rewarded, other behaviour is discouraged. It's everyday life, in other words. We give our children gifts or rewards when they are "good," and scold or punish them when they are "bad." Teachers give stars for good work and time out for misbehaviour. Why in the world would psychiatrists practise something so ordinary? Aren't they embarrassed to realize they've become highly paid personal trainers?

My assumption has always been that psychiatry enters people's lives only when things are seriously amiss and ordinary methods have failed. When parents, social-support systems, and schools find their methods ineffective, something else is called for, and a psychiatrist is called in. But behaviour modification, despite famous behaviourists like Pavlov and Skinner, is ordinary.

Patients treated with IPT are encouraged to have normal human interactions. Who, I demand to know, decides which behaviours are normal? If I'm a loner, "not fit for human company," as I often say of myself, whose business is it but mine? These methods are a swindle, although that word is too polite. Really it's social engineering.

✣ ✣ ✣

Freud once made a politically incorrect joke about women, the type still (quietly) made by men, including male doctors. Politically adroit, Freud disclaimed authorship of the joke, saying he was quoting someone else. Nevertheless, in talking of hysterics, Freud offered this prescription:

> *Rx*
> *Penis normalis*
> *Dosum: repetatur*

[Take thou of . . . et cetera.]

Men's sexist jokes are traditionally made in the company of other men. I don't have access to the jokes made by women about men, but I suspect equivalent sexist jokes bubble away merrily in the world of women. There is a point to such jokes. Freud meant that the refreshment and awakening of gender identity cures women — men, too — and sexual activity has precisely such a ceremonial effect. When he theorized about sexual drives, Freud forgot the symbolic/ceremonial part, but showed he knew better when he later confessed that drives are a psychoanalytic myth. I also know that men, pathetic on their own, are expected to do better if hooked up with a good woman.

Like many modern psychiatrists, some of Freud's colleagues forgot their task was to analyze crippling symbolic messages. Instead, they thought friendliness was the key to helping people. I'm not sure how they came to the conclusion — which they believed — that their friendliness was better than that of others; perhaps their high fees convinced them their personal qualities must be worth the price. Freud took his friend and colleague Sandor Ferenczi to task.[1]

You have not made a secret of the fact that you kiss your patients and let them kiss you. . . . I am assuredly not one of those who from prudishness or bourgeois convention condemn little erotic gratifications of this kind. . . . We have hitherto in our technique held to the conclusion that patients are to be refused erotic gratifications. . . . Now picture what will be the result of publishing your technique. There is no revolutionary who is not driven out of the field by a still more radical one. A number of independent thinkers in matters of technique will say to themselves: why stop at a kiss? Certainly one gets further when one adopts "pawing" as well, which after all doesn't make a baby. And then bolder ones will come along who will go further, to peeping and showing — and soon we shall have accepted in the technique of analysis all the tricks of *demi-viergerie* and petting parties. . . . and God the Father Ferenczi gazing at the lively scene he has created will perhaps say to himself: maybe after all I should have halted in my technique of motherly affection before the kiss. . . .

Ferenczi acted foolishly, as did the doctor I've just read about in my professional college's discipline-committee publication. When this family doctor's patient wanted to masturbate, as a therapeutic tactic he squatted beside her, observed carefully, and made detailed notes for his records of what he observed. Among other things, he noted that the patient's attachment to him had become sexualized and added — again in his notes — that he himself was not aroused. What does this illustrate? That human folly, be it preposterously rationalized sexuality or ordinary kisses, can always be made to seem reasonable?

I'm sure Ferenczi felt better when he gave little kisses; improved or consolidated his image of himself as a kind doctor. I'd also guess he didn't kiss his male patients, which, as Freud tells him, suggests a heterosexual erotic factor. Plainly said, he was using his patients to lay in a bit of extra male confidence for himself. No harm in that, I say, except not with patients, who have fulfilled their responsibilities to us once they've paid the bill. We all use our patients for our own vain purposes, but if we're doing our job, we busily worry about this, hoping to read and restrain our own secret purposes. Patients have no responsibility to pump up the psychiatrist's gender identity. Best if Ferenczi had followed the advice in this advertisement from a recent edition of the *Globe and Mail* newspaper:

> MBH is unlike anything else because it's not a drug that can cause dangerous, unhealthy side effects. It's an all-natural, scientifically-formulated blend of the highest potency herbs that work with the male biochemistry to help heighten your sex drive and give you back your youthful sexual stamina and sexual ability. MBH users say they not only increase their stamina and performance level, they also achieve stronger, longer-lasting erections, maximizing sexual pleasure and satisfaction.

✢ ✢ ✢

The woman with the squeal got me thinking. I remembered that, when I joked with the woman on the bicycle beside me about what I'd seen, I'd had the fleeting thought she might denounce me for making a sexist remark. She'd smiled, so I'd not misjudged her, but it reminded me of a difficult occasion when I met with an investigator at the College of Physicians and Surgeons of Ontario. A woman had made a complaint about me concerning some imagined misconduct — and the investigator, speaking to my lawyer in my presence, referred to me as a "sex-abuse case."

Later, unsettled and angry, I commented on the remark to my lawyer. I straightened my shoulders and held my head high in mock pride: "Well, I didn't know I was a sex-abuse case!" In other words, I clearly reasserted my male potency — not because I'd abused someone, but because of the investigator's jargon — and felt better.

✢ ✢ ✢

Good psychiatrists focus on stories like that of the young woman who squealed, tiny events from everyday life. We remind ourselves that "the devil is in the details." Psychiatrists also know how to target big rituals, the traditional cultural ceremonies devised to nail down maleness and womanliness.

✛ ✛ ✛

In 1988, three friends and I came upon a crowd of people outside of a village near the townships of Cape Town. I was frightened, because I thought it was a riot. Many young men were yelling and fighting. Once we got close, however, I saw this was semi-organized sport. The boys — they were teenagers — had thick towels or blankets wrapped around their left arms, and with their right arms, swung hard and viciously at one another with staves. They hit out with all their might, aiming, it seemed, to injure one another. Then I noticed a group of younger boys, also fighting with sticks, although they yelled and laughed because they were playing, and their game was innocent fun. The older boys, serious about their fighting, were silent.

Our driver in the Cape Town townships told us the older boys had just come down from the mountains, where, for a few days, they'd fasted and taken hallucinogenic drugs, been shown secret grottos, and then been circumcised. Now, men at last, they had become adult warriors. The younger boys, I realized, were playfully copying them, rehearsing for the day when they, too, would go up to the mountains.

Our African driver didn't add that, when these young men played war, they were doing the same as me when I criticize my colleagues. Do you remember the poison dart in my (polite) statement in Chapter 3 that "When cornered, biological psychiatrists admit nothing has been discovered . . ."? The African boys didn't have to offer their knuckles to be rapped with a scalpel by someone like J. C. Boileau Grant, my professor of anatomy, nor did they dissect cadavers, or go through the hell of anatomy, but they did the equivalent. We call the rituals of

Africans primitive and superstitious. What a laugh! Like a curmud-
geonly warrior, I've now mocked every reader who thought the African
boys were superstitious.

But the celebration of manhood is ambivalent. I've seen African
dancers, all men, dancing "women's dances," which women were not
allowed to perform. The men weren't, like drag-queens, caricaturing
women, so I was taken aback at their womanliness.

In the West, a hundred years ago, it was common for male infants
and toddlers to wear dresses and to have long ringlets. The shearing
of ringlets was popularly recognized as a time for a mother to shed
tears. I remember having to (gently) insist on my eldest son's first
haircut, which I administered. That haircut was clearly ceremonial,
thrilling, and important. The feminization of young men has a long
history; teachers in ancient Greece insisted on the intensely erotic
nature of inspirational teaching: homosexual love between teacher
and student was highly acclaimed. Only the intrusion of hairy legs
brought bliss to an end.

I've heard another explanation of the feminization of boys: it's the
evil eye. If the birth of a male child isn't kept quiet, I was told, the evil
eye will be envious, so it's smart (wink, wink) to keep it under your hat
if a son is born. My patient Yang Keyuan confirmed that this happens
in Chinese culture, too. If a male baby has died, the birth of sons born
later is kept secret, just in case. Celebration of manhood should be
deferred until the boy is safely an adult.

Preventive medicine is available: if the machinations of the evil eye
are a serious risk, do like Catholics and Hindus in Goa: consult a wise
woman. She will sprinkle salt and guide you as you toss a few chilies
into a fire. If they explode, you'll be fine. The old woman may even have
a tip for you; if your crops are lush, hang a skull in a tree near the field.
This will nicely ward off the envious evil eye.

Homer told the following story first (did *The Iliad* anticipate everything?). Achilles the fleet-of-foot, greatest of runners, was the
quintessential male hero. No masculine figure could, or will, surpass
him. And yet, he was raised as a girl, his maleness a secret, distinguished

only by the brusque way he tossed back his hair. Despite secrecy, out of their passion, he and Daidameia, one of the girls with whom he was raised, had a child: Neoptolemus.

‡ ‡ ‡

Every telling story is personal. Even the most profound have been understood, albeit vaguely, when we are children. Dona was my mother's sister, and when she stayed over, she slept in my bed. I noticed her negligee, probably silk, because in 1939 nylon and polyester hadn't yet been invented. I also noticed a smell. I wasn't sure it was a bad smell, but I didn't like it. It was too intimate and too personal. My young mind may have had other thoughts, but my way of remembering the scene is that the smell came from her skin. Since we are stereotypically German, I know she would have been fastidiously clean; she was fussier than my mother. But my sexually alert mind was nervous about the whole business.

A few years later, in 1942, I overheard Dona and my mother talking. Although I didn't fully understand, the gist was that, when Dona had a regular sex life, her vagina was healthy; when she was without a lover, she had a discharge. (Do you remember my gynecology professor who said, "The vagina is a self-cleansing organ"?) My mother and aunt spoke in German, of course, and even today I have no idea how the vagina is referred to in colloquial German. But I do remember a word, a peculiar word spoken in an outlandish dialect, a mixture of Swiss and Austrian peasant dialects. To my ears it was disturbingly intimate, lowbrow, childlike, vulgar. The word was *Füdele*. It conjures in my mind the quivering lips of a dark, moist vagina.

I recently asked a German friend, who has no background of village dialects, about the word. He'd never heard it, but screwed up his face and admitted that, without understanding the word, it conjured up something vaguely unsettling. I understood; it still unsettles *me*.

There was another word associated with this overheard conversation that was even more disturbing. This time it was a respectable German word that I knew well: *Eiter*. It means "pus." My Aunt Dona, when without a sexual life, had gobs of pus coming out of her vagina — I thought.

The last instalment of this story took place fifteen years later. I was an intern at the Vancouver General Hospital, and Dona lived in Vancouver. That I was a doctor meant to her that she could speak frankly. "*Weiss' du*," she said, "*dass wenn ich nicht mit'n Mann bin, kommt mir Eiter von der Vagina?* (Do you know that when I'm not with a man, pus comes out of my vagina?)"

She didn't know how to say it like a psychiatrist: when she and a man perform the ceremonies of love, she is transformed into a woman, and her somatic troubles end.

✛ ✛ ✛

Something that defines a woman comes out of the vagina: blood. Anita Diamant's novel *The Red Tent*[2] tells how, each month, women in ancient Israel moved into a red tent for a few days or a week. Like Persephone, they'd bitten the pomegranate — the apple of maturity — spilled its blood-red juice, and become fertile. With the onset of menses, they were given access to the red tent. For those so honoured it was a special time; women who did not bleed — those who were pre-pubertal and post-menopausal — brought food, bathed the women in the tent, and stroked their skin. In compliance with this important destiny, to this day women and girls who live in close quarters in camps or dormitories perform this defining act in unison; girls who live together bleed at the same time or, also together, decline to menstruate at all.

Women don't identify only with one another; they identify with the actual bleeding activities of their bodies. This story from the Koran — it doesn't appear in the Judeo-Christian Bible — illustrates the symbolic importance of blood:

Joseph, her beautiful slave-boy, had enthralled Potiphar's wife. Because her friends were baffled that a lady of her rank would sink to loving a slave, she invited her friends to tea. She served fresh pears and apples and, to cut the fruit, made sure each guest had a beautiful and sharp silver knife. Potiphar's wife arranged for Joseph to enter the room at the moment they were serving themselves. What Potiphar's wife expected indeed happened: when her friends — ladies-in-waiting, hangers-on, minor nobility — cut their fruit, Joseph's beauty so took them aback that they cut their fingers to the bone. The carnage was awful, the room spattered with blood. The sight of the beautiful slave-boy had awakened their identification with their own bleeding genitals. Potiphar's wife was a shrewd psychologist.

CHAPTER NINE

DECENCY, VIRTUE, RIGHTEOUSNESS

WHEN I FIRST READ TOLSTOY'S SHORT STORY "The Kreutzer Sonata," I admired it. Although my admiration has not faded, I now know things about the writing of the story that shock me. It concerns a conversation between strangers on a train, one of whom tells how, in a fit of jealousy, he murdered his innocent wife. The man, Pózdnyshev, attributes his jealousy to social factors; the Russian and European cultures' encouragement of lechery, a degeneracy that has infected most of the public. He argues that, not only should licentiousness be brought to an end, but even marital congress avoided.

Pózdnyshev is a madman, a moralist beyond belief, not to speak of his cowardly conviction that social circumstances make him innocent of the murder of his wife. Had he not been indoctrinated to lust by Russian culture, he says, the murder would not have happened.

Pózdnyshev is bizarre. His arguments, although logical, are grounded in a morality so arbitrary and severe that he is nothing less than a wild-eyed loony. The fascination of the story is, to me, Tolstoy's even-handed portrait, allowing the character to flesh out his mad beliefs without moralizing. I'm not Tolstoy, and could never describe a cruel, harsh-minded moralist without tossing in a bit of counter-moralizing of my own. Since I'm in a non-moralizing profession, this is an embarrassing confession.

Tolstoy wrote an afterword to "The Kreutzer Sonata," explaining what he'd intended by the story. I was astonished to find I'd been dead wrong. Tolstoy wasn't intending to caricature a moral monster; he was of the same opinion as Pózdnyshev. He believed marital intimacy was filth and moral disease, and should be abandoned.

> In order for men not to behave this way, it is necessary that . . . *both before and after marriage* they would not regard falling in love and the carnal love connected with it as a poetic and elevated state as they look on it now, but rather as a state of bestiality degrading for a human being. . . . abstinence, which constitutes a necessary condition of human dignity during the period of the unmarried state, *is even more necessary in marriage itself.* [my italics]

One of my personal cures, a placebo that turns my crank, is disagreement, sometimes disguised. Most people hate being called conventional, and it stings when we are told we've uttered a cliché. Many more are disappointed when a favourite restaurant, the one no one else knows about, becomes fashionable. But I'm a terminal case of oppositionalism: I can't enjoy a book acclaimed as one the greatest of European novels, *War and Peace*. I like *Anna Karenina* and Tolstoy's short stories, but to me Tolstoy's magnum opus is a disappointment, wrecked by the same moralizing that, in "The Kreutzer Sonata," makes it so bizarre. It's no secret that in his personal life Tolstoy was sadistic, a sexual libertine, and an ignoble fool, so it's remarkable that, when describing fictional events, he is dispassionate, descriptive, and discerning. That's what makes him great.

Those who, like me, often disagree with others, and devote themselves to finding error — wickedness — in others, have discovered the most effective cure for the woes of life. It's the "external devil" trick. This defensive style is one of the great afflictions of mankind — except it's a deed and not an affliction against which we are powerless. It's a device all of us use, mostly because it's easy to divide by two: bad and good. "Either/or" is easy; "and/or" demands mental work. We daren't, like Pózdnyshev, blame our culture; were it trendy to dislike Tolstoy, Aboriginal people, or Jews, we'd still have a choice about signing up with popular opinion.

I'm pretty good at noticing when I blame others — or so I think — but the truth is that, although I make the right noises, I'm as guilty of it as everyone else. Because this offence never ends, as psychiatrists do their work, introspection will always be their first priority. I wish the evil of blaming came back to haunt us, but to believe this is to believe in a fairy tale. Since we're all expert at deciding the other guy is wrong, self-righteous blaming will always be endemic. It's the disease of which it claims to be the cure.

Another kind of man, Odysseus, was not one-sided: he was the man of twists and turns, a wily tactician, traveller, and loyal husband. When the Achaeans were preparing for war, he tried to avoid being drafted and, donning "the headgear of a madman," planted salt in the furrows of his fields instead of seeds. Rather than shouting his approval of the Greek attack on the Trojans, he was unsure of the Greek cause. In his few appearances in the pages of *The Iliad*, Odysseus isn't seen hacking at the heads and limbs of Trojans; in a cunning disguise he walks the streets of Troy, meets and talks to Helen, but later is prominent among those hidden in the hollow horse.

✢✢✢

The following case report is not a classical example of blaming; I've already given one: "The Kreutzer Sonata." And in the psychiatric clinic, the obvious blamers — of parents, bosses, doctors, trauma, and disease — are all too common. The patient I have in mind is a more ordinary fellow. But Mr. Tony Burke, whom I saw a few years ago in a seminar with psychiatric students, was preoccupied by virtue. This was no particular surprise, because virtue enters into the psychological balance of every case. Indeed, it enters into the psychological balance of every one of us. This young man brought the issue to life in his own way; like Tolstoy, he impoverished himself by trying to find sexiness and "dirty thinking" only in others.

Dr. Fahima Sadiq, a new student, had no licence to practise medicine in Canada. Like a number of foreign graduates, she attended my seminar so she could add Canadian credentials to her curriculum vitae. Such students enjoy the seminar but, since most of them are qualified doctors in their own country, it's a humiliation to be *obliged* to be a student again. For their work, they earn the right to say that they served an externship with me. This was the first case she'd presented, so the other students and I were curious. Since she'd had no psychiatric training (apart from sitting in on my seminar for a couple of months), I was ready for the worst.

The other students around the table — there were seven or eight of them — were alert. They were gearing up to assign Dr. Sadiq to a place in the hierarchy.

Mike Marconi, a non-medical trainee in one of Toronto's psychoanalytic institutes, was attending the seminar for a second year. At first I'd found him silly; although smart, he wore black leather and had earrings, and his lank hair fell below his shoulders. This attire was garnished with a heavy chain, laden with keys that looped from belt to pocket. This was risky attire in the formal world of CAMH, but his intelligence allowed him to get away with it. I'd come to like him better; he no longer had a knee-jerk argumentative reaction to me. I'd never argued back and my amused smiles — secretly smug — seemed to have disarmed him.

Like all our choices, Mike's attire was his self-cure, proof that he was no boring conformist. In other words, placebo cures are both ordinary and profound, and when doctors accomplish them, they accomplish what all of us do all the time. Our ways are solutions to the problems of living. I frequently remind the students that psychiatric problems are not problems after all; they are the solution. Madness isn't mad; it is one man's shrewd answer. The problems that matter are hidden.

Hidden problems are discovered after arduous work, and turn out not to be the "real" problem either. Behind every answer is another answer, and behind that, yet another. There's a story told in India in which a Colonel Blimp figure, an English colonialist, was told that the world rests on the back of an elephant.

"What," he asked, "does the elephant stand on?"

The Indian man he was talking to replied, "On the back of a turtle."

"And what does the turtle stand on?"

"On another turtle, Sahib."

Enthralled as he was by his rationality-madness, his Aristotelian metaphysics, and demanding of himself and the storyteller literal rather than poetic truth, the Englishman had no choice but to ask again, "And what does *that* turtle stand on?"

"Ah, Sahib," said the Indian, "from there on, it's turtles all the way down."

What we psychiatrists unearth is never a resting point, only a variant. None of us seems able to get the wonderful truth about "the meaning of life" through our heads.

"Mr. Tony Burke is twenty-nine," said Dr. Sadiq. "He's a computer programmer, but studied physics and got a graduate degree before deciding to change course. He couldn't explain why he gave up physics, but he didn't do much for a year and then went to college to study computers.

"He says he has obsessions about women. He's had a number of relationships with women, but most weren't really girlfriends. He falls in love and then becomes preoccupied with a woman, even if he's never spoken to her. He's also obsessed by the *idea* of women, and thinks about them all the time, women that don't exist. He fell in love with his boss and decided he had to do something, so he told her. Apparently she became annoyed and said she wasn't interested.

"He's nice-looking, not creepy like the story sounds, and doesn't look insecure either. His boss is his age and single, and till then they'd been good friends, so I'm not sure why she would have been annoyed. Next, he fell in love with a woman he met with friends from George Brown College. She was French, and when she went back to Nice, he quit his job and went to be with her. They went out for a while, but then broke up and he came back to Canada.

"He always picks someone close to his friends or family. The way he describes it, other people put him together with these women, as though it's an accident, or that he didn't have anything to do with it. Once he was obsessed by a friend of his mother's, and then with a friend of his aunt's. I think he went out with them once or twice and then stopped.

"He says his family is nice. His father is a car mechanic with his own shop and makes a good living. The father is quiet and his mother is the boss. She works, too, but I forgot to ask what she did.

"He has no brothers or sisters. He grew up in Etobicoke and was an above-average student. He always had friends and played sports, but didn't go out with girls while in school.

"Oh, yes. One more thing. He says he saw you when he was a child. The chart didn't come up until just before he arrived, so I haven't had a chance to see what was going on when you saw him."

I was pleased by Dr. Sadiq's good presentation; she neither used jargon nor looked anxiously at me as she spoke, checking for approval. She was self-confident and had made astute observations. *Once she's had formal psychiatric training, she'll lapse into jargon*, I thought. *She doesn't know that her plain language has brought the patient to life, and once she catches on to the local lingo, she'll be less interesting.*

She hadn't read the chart, but it sat on the conference table in front of her. I didn't want to teach the students bad habits, imply to them that reviewing the chart had priority over seeing the patient, so I turned to Dr. Sadiq and said, "Could you please bring Mr. Burke in?" She picked up the chart and, as she passed by, handed it to me.

As I stood waiting for the patient to arrive, I glanced at the chart lying in front of me on the table. It easily opened to the note I'd written twenty-two years before. I read a few lines, closed the chart, and shoved it back on the table. I'd instantly remembered the case.

I didn't remember four-year-old Tony Burke, but I remembered his mother. She'd been attractive, with high colour and a fine bosom. I'd

liked her. She was worried about Tony's thumb-sucking. But it wasn't
as simple as that; the habit was complex. He had a security blanket
that, like Linus, he carried with him, held either against his crotch or
his cheek. Most days, he would pee in his pants, just enough to make a
wet patch and to create a wet patch on his blanket. He'd then hold the
warm, wet part of his blanket tight against his cheek with one hand,
clutch the wet patch on his pants with the other, then suck lustily on
his thumb. That day, twenty-two years later, I couldn't recall the exact
mechanics, but what I remembered would have required him to have
three hands.

Mrs. Burke hadn't said so explicitly, but like me, she'd sensed this
complex symptom cluster was masturbatory, unique, and designed for
Tony's own purposes: a personal self-curative ceremony. "He's so sensual," she'd said. "I remember when he was a baby, he'd suck the
breast so excitedly. I thought it was wonderful, but now I'm wondering
if he wasn't overdoing it."

I remember looking at Mrs. Burke, acutely aware of how sensual
she was. I wondered to myself when it was that Tony Burke had
retreated from sensual interest to erotic coolness.

But I didn't tell this 1980 story to the students, because I feared
they'd fall into a trap. Enthralled by the theory of causality, they'd think
that, because the mother was sensual, she'd *caused* the boy to have
sexual problems. They'd get the rest of the story straight, that Mr.
Burke was excitedly sensual when he obsessed and thought frantically
about women, and another side of him fought this off: he couldn't get
connected with a woman, despite his obsessive preoccupation.
Instead, the students, up-and-coming parent-bashers all, would use
my secret story to persuade themselves that Mr. Burke's complaints
were the fault of his mother. So I held my tongue. That ancient history
was to be *my* secret. No harm having a leg up on the students.

Dr. Sadiq opened the door and came in, followed by Mr. Burke.
"This is Dr. Warme," she said.

I stepped forward and shook his hand: "How do you do?" I said.

"Hi," he replied.

I sat quietly. It's good not to be a chatterbox. Best to let the patient start thinking. He was nervous and I saw he was hoping I'd have a list of questions to which he could give concrete answers, information like "yes," "no," or, "in 1991."

"You fall deeply in love, I hear."

"Love?" he said, looking worried. He was thinner than I'd expected. His shirt was too big and, because he pushed his shoulders forward, his chest looked hollow.

I waited again. In interviews, an atmosphere of uncertainty is important. It peaks curiosity, keeps patients thinking, and makes me mysterious. "Yes, in love. Again and again."

"I don't fall in love; I obsess about women," he announced emphatically. I noted that, in his first remarks, eroticism was attributed to me, not him: by using the word "love" I'd been sexy; by saying "obsess" he'd stuck with safe, clinical language. Virtue was in the air.

I gave a tiny smile, barely perceptible. "It seems to me one of the main things about love is that, when it happens, we get obsessed, don't we?"

His eyes opened wider. He felt caught.

"You look so amazed," I said, "as though I'd caught you. I'm not sure why that would make you uncomfortable. Seems to me, falling in love is one of the commonest things on the planet."

"Uh, it's just that, when it happens, I'm so obsessed. I lie in bed and think about the woman. It's crazy."

"The madness of love, perhaps? I guess whoever said it was right: 'love is folly.'" I waited for thirty to forty seconds till he could get his breath back and his thinking on track, and then added, "Lost in love. Yeah, that's what it is, lost in love."

"Well, sort of," he answered. "But really it's that I think about them all the time."

"Isn't that what being in love is like? Being lost in it?"

He looked puzzled, "That would be crazy."

"So you don't like to get lost. Actually, I have another word I like: yield. You don't like to yield to love."

"I see what you mean, but . . ."

"I'm going to tell you a story," I said. "It's the story of Echo and Narcissus.

"Echo got into trouble with Hera, the queen of Olympus. Zeus had been involved in hanky-panky with some nymph, and Echo kept his secret, so Hera was furious. The punishment she imposed on Echo was that she would lose her speech, except to repeat the last few words of what other people had just said. You know, like an echo in a chamber or a valley.

"Anyway, it came to pass that Echo fell in love with Narcissus, a handsome young man. She couldn't speak to him, of course, but she followed him around. If Narcissus had spoken, she wouldn't have been able to reply, except to repeat his last three or four words. Narcissus didn't like Echo's pursuit, and tried to get away. Finally, he spoke to her emphatically:

"'*Never*,' he said, 'will I yield to you!'

"And Echo replied, softly, 'I *yield* to you.'

"Mr. Burke, I love telling stories, and I could pile on a few more about yielding, like the story of stubborn old King Lear and his stubborn daughter Cordelia, both of whom eventually yielded, but that will have to wait. I think you understand the point I'm making when I tell the story of Echo and Narcissus, right?"

"Yeah, I guess you're right. I don't like to yield."

"Have you ever had sex with a woman, Mr. Burke?"

"No sir, I haven't," he replied.

"What about masturbation? Are you able to masturbate?"

This may seem like impropriety, asking personal questions in front of an audience. But I could see that, suddenly, Mr. Burke had become lost in the interview — he'd *yielded* to the interview — and hardly knew the students were there. I, too, was lost in the interview. Both of us leaned forward just a bit, my mouth slightly open, his the opposite, lips tightly pursed. There was electricity in the air, and a fantasy: perhaps Mr. Burke's crinkly hair would shed sparks.

"Uh, yes, I masturbate."

"What fantasies do you have while masturbating?"

"Oh, just girls I know."

"What kind of girls? Do you have to submit to them, yield to them, in other words?"

I confess. I had a leg up on the students, because I'd once known his mother and was aware of his childhood history. If I'd convinced the students I was a wizard, no harm would have been done; students need wizardly teachers. I'd offered the idea that, when masturbating, he might have had an interest in submitting to women because of his history — that, as a boy, he might have imagined he had to submit to the sensuality of his mother, and that he might repeat this in his masturbatory life. But my hunch was wrong.

"Oh, no. It's not like that at all. I like to have fantasies of *young* women."

His comment silenced me for a moment, but it was my duty to perform, to create a bit of pedagogical theatre for the students. As I watched Mr. Burke's doubts and fears, I realized I'd have to coach him a bit more.

"Oh, the women are young, are they? Not well developed? Slim hips and small breasts, perhaps?"

"Yeah, that's the kind of women I have fantasies about. I don't have to submit to them."

"They're not fully developed, then?" Mr. Burke had spent an hour being interviewed by Dr. Sadiq. If he was uneasy about mature women, he would have noticed Dr. Sadiq had an attractive, full figure. I didn't wait for his answer.

"To get lost in love, or lost in a fully developed woman, isn't exactly to your taste?"

He responded with a weak quibble. "Well, I'm not sure I'd go that far."

"The women in your fantasies are young and not voluptuous, so you don't have to worry about them being enthusiastically alive, sexually alive. They're probably sort of gentle and sweet. But if you had a fantasy about a highly sexed women, she'd sort of take you by surprise, catch you off guard. Such a woman would be unpredictable and, if you yielded to her, you'd be all full of nervousness. I wonder if that's why you don't like to yield?

"Something else. I notice that you often quibble when I say something, maybe even get a bit stubborn. I think that's the same thing; you don't like to yield to me either. You have a graduate degree in physics, I believe. I'll bet you didn't like Heisenberg's Uncertainty Principle much?"

He responded with another quibble. "Yeah, but that's not really physics."

I narrowed my eyes. Mr. Burke blushed. He'd noticed his fear of yielding to new ideas, my penetrations, and most important, yielding to my erotic intimacy with his secrets.

"But you only quibbled about the Heisenberg Principle. I guess that means you agree with me that mature women make you uneasy?"

His eyes were wide open and he looked pale.

"Mr. Burke," I said, "it's time to stop. We'll find someone for you to work with. Dr. Sadiq will give you a call."

Mr. Burke had cured himself with virtue, the cure he now called a problem. He certainly didn't, like the girl in Chapter 8 who became more feminine, celebrate his gender. She, you'll remember, saved herself by squealing. Mr. Burke had devised the opposite cure: killing his own maleness, being uninterested in women who were erotically enthusiastic, did the trick. He was good, pure and clean; fully feminine women were, in his mind, frighteningly arousing, probably dirty pigs. His virtue solution, a personal ceremony of living, was to think — dryly, repetitively, and unproductively. He was an obsessive — a dry stick, in other words. He politely got up and walked out of the room.

There was tension in the room, but it no longer leached out of Mr. Burke; now it was in the students. They were troubled by my brusqueness. I'd made them think. Because they thought I should have given Mr. Burke reassurance and encouragement, they were most bothered most at the end of the interview. But that's not my style. I'd have felt I was patronizing him, uttering platitudes.

✢ ✢ ✢

Louise, one of the less-fearful students, spoke up. "Why would he be so afraid of women? You often bring that up when you interview men."

While living her life, Lou hadn't been paying attention. Actually, it's more likely she didn't want to *admit* that she'd paid attention and perfectly well knew the answer to her own question. Like all of us, she'd heard the jokes, made by both men and women, about the smelly vagina: "fishy," is how it's described. This is a tricky topic, not politically correct perhaps: I'm supposed to reassure the students that such fantasies, rather than being universal, are a silly prejudice.

When I tell students my secret thoughts about such topics, I'm greeted by bafflement. I'm baffled, too, partly because I can't figure out why they don't enjoy thought experiments. *For crying out loud,* I think to myself, *my patients listen to such talk with interest.* Or is it that my patients are brainwashed, sucked in by me, rendered in thrall to a heroic image of me, the doctor who can do no wrong? Some mad transference reaction I don't have the guts or intelligence to analyze?

The ancient Greeks — who discovered everything, and in their mythic cosmology talked about everything — neglected the anxious thoughts we all have just as Lou did, or at least neglected explicit mention of it. The primal example is Medusa, the beautiful woman who incurred the enmity of Athena by lying with Poseidon in Athena's shrine. Medusa's punishment? Her hair thickened, the tips became serpent's heads, and she grew into the horrible Medusa of the snaky locks.

Sexiness, especially with senior gods like Poseidon (earth-shaker, brother of Zeus and Hades, king of the sea, one of the three great realms of the universe), is a big crime. Since Poseidon is one of the fathers, it's an incestuous/Oedipal crime. Athena therefore imposed a severe penalty. In contrast to Medusa, because they'd committed no sins, Cinderella and Snow White became beautiful; Medusa was a sinner, so became ugly and revolting, the element in the story that would have suited Mr. Burke perfectly. And when Perseus hacked off Medusa's head, even Homer and the Greek playwrights wouldn't or couldn't say that the stump of Medusa's neck was a vagina. I've already mentioned that, at the instant her head was lopped off, the stump gave birth to Pegasus and Chrysaor. Like Lou, the Greek writers didn't want to acknowledge what they knew.

I stay quiet when students ask nervous questions, which I explain by saying I want them to think for themselves, that I won't patronize them by knowing all the answers. This behaviour weaves a cloak of mystery. *How else*, I tell myself, *am I to be a teaching influence?* These are my conscious thoughts, the reasons and causes I conjure up to make sense of my behaviour. The best truth, a difficult one, is to say, "This is how I teach." And is the need for a cloak of mystery the reason why both we and the ancient Greek myths are vague about the details of the sexual imagination?

But I *want* to answer Lou's questions. *Men are easy to figure out, Lou,* I want to say. *They have a penis, easy to see, which raises only simple questions. Although I'm going to say this in an amusing way, it's serious and important. What are the questions? Well, does the penis stand up or does it not stand up? Does it squirt or does it not squirt? And that's about it.*

The other students would watch intently. Even though he wouldn't succeed in hiding his scorn for my methods, Mike would act as though I were giving medical information and busily take notes. Others would do something similar, catalogue my words for use on some examination. Privately, some would think I was nuts, especially the ones who think suffering is cured by love. Those whom I've brainwashed would gasp at my effrontery. Others still, those as baffled as me, would think and learn – or so says my biased tyranny.

A woman's genital is another matter, I would go on. *It's a complicated organ, never clearly seen. It's hidden and internal. The vagina is dark and mysterious, has secret nooks and crannies, unknown even to women, the possessors of vaginas. And, Lou, it also has an ambiguous smell. We all know about the revulsion at the smell of the vagina, but we also know — I don't think we talk about this — that its smell is attractive. It's the place of mystery.*

That's why Mr. Burke has trouble with women. He hates mysteries and wants everything clear. And that's why I guessed he wouldn't like Heisenberg's Uncertainty Principle. The same goes for Relativity Theory. He likes to pin things down, and when I got vague or allusive, he quibbled and tried to argue.

Young women, women without breasts, hips and buttocks, are barely acceptable, but sexual women, in other words those with vaginas, are disturbing. The glistening radiance of a real woman is to be avoided.

But, either a sage or a coward, I held my tongue. *I can't believe I'm being politically correct,* I thought.

Dr. Warme, Lou would say, *you're the only person in the world I know who would talk that way.*

Are you an idiot or something? I would answer. *How can I be a psychiatrist if I don't speak frankly? Such talk isn't the stuff of dinner-party conversation, but we, the experts, have no choice.*

✦ ✦ ✦

There were other ideas in the air that day, indiscreet, provocative, possibly even true: simple penises and complex vaginas are connected to the differing roles of men and women in disturbing the peace of the world. When a man commits rape, everything is turned upside down; the woman's marriage and family are destabilized, the order of things changed forever. Think of Achilles, Hector, Tony Soprano. Warriors wipe out confidence in virgin daughters, loyal wives, protective fathers, and husbands. The world is shattered and must be reinvented.

According to the ancients, women change the world through betrayal. The adulterous wife destabilizes marriage and family, and undoes the order of things: Emma Bovary, Anna Karenina, Helen of Troy. We don't give a damn (well, we do a bit) about husbands who betray; only a woman, through adultery, has the power to force the world to be reinvented.

Like a penis, rape is simple and obvious; like a vagina, adultery is mysterious and secret. In the chief non-dominant gender culture, homosexuality, the theme and variations are less stereotypical, harder for a heterosexual psychiatrist to figure out. But typically, only by learning about the mysteries of women can a man become wise like Odysseus. And only by learning about the bold actions of Zeus can a woman become tough and confident like Athena. Of all the gods, she was the only one allowed to use Zeus' thunderbolt.

✦ ✦ ✦

The students are naive; some don't even know young children masturbate. Nor do they realize that dreams and sex are special. All too quickly, a man who complains of impotence gets a prescription for Viagra or one of its newer cousins. They don't ask the obvious, either because their training has failed them, or — probably it's the same thing — because all cultures practise sexual privacy. But doctors aren't just nice; the culture has designated them to do unusual things. Were the students not so circumspect they would ask, "Who are you impotent with?"

The answer is in this story from Hermann Kurzke's biography *Thomas Mann: Life as a Work of Art*, a classical story of the self-cure through blaming.[1] Thomas Mann had developed the story from a few lines in the *Malleus Maleficarum*.

In Merssburg near Constance there lived toward the end of the fifteenth century an honest lad named Heinz Klöpfgeissel, a cooper by trade, of good stature and health. He had an intimate interrelationship with a girl, Bärbel, the only daughter of a widowed bell ringer, and wanted to marry her, but the wishes of the pair met paternal resistance, for Klöpfgeissel was a poor fellow and the bell ringer first demanded a goodly position in life from him, that he become a master in his trade before he would give him his daughter. But the affections of the young people were stronger than their patience, and the pair had already turned into a couple. For at night, when the bell ringer had gone bell ringing, Klöpfgeissel climbed in to Bärbel, and their embraces made each one seem to the other the most glorious thing on earth.

But one day he and other young companions were feeling their oats, and they decided to go to women in a sporting house. But there his otherwise sturdy erection failed, and also a second time, when he found a landlady willing, his flesh would not rise. Only with his Bärbel, while the bell ringer was bell ringing, did he further have the most successful hours. That he could do it only with a single person, left him in no doubt any longer that he was bewitched [he blamed his imagined impotence on betwitchment]; he confides to a priest, who notifies the Inquisition of the case; Bärbel confesses and is burned at the stake. Heinz Klöpfgeissel, the bewitched man, stood with a bare head, murmuring prayers in the mass of spectators.

What the students don't know is that, apart from rare cases of impotence due to medical causes, impotence is selective, as is premature ejaculation, failure of orgasm, and unwanted frequent orgasm. One woman, anorgasmic with her husband, was troubled because, like thunderbolts flung from the arm of Zeus, repeated orgasms shuddered through her when she walked past an attractive male colleague. Men and women alike desire, awaken, and discharge selectively.

Some are sexually competent with those they love, others never with those they love. Women incapable of arousal in the marital bed sometimes fall in love, leave their husbands, and become sexually vivacious. Others, although bored and passionless, function as dependably with their spouses as a Rolex watch. But only if naughty or in a compromising situation are they desirous and thrilled. Some men, with kaleidoscopic variety, are more sexual with young women or old, with prostitutes or with children, with other men or with corpses. Sexual preference and plasticity is infinite.

The question rarely asked by students — "Who are you impotent with?" — isn't important because it will lead to a cure for this or that sexual dysfunction; it will help them familiarize their patient with who he or she is. The courageous acknowledgement of the shifting variety of sexual styles advances intelligent conversation.

CHAPTER TEN

FIRM CONVICTION

SCIENCE AND REASON ARE *MY* PLACEBO CURE. They don't relieve symptoms or wounds, nor do they cure me of disease or folly; yet they are the rod and the staff that comfort me and restore my soul.

My attachment to Science and Reason also reveals what I'm tempted to believe: if people would think well, pull themselves together, use their heads, the world would be a better place. Because this view includes the idea that disciplined thinking makes for a disciplined world — as though it's obvious this would be a good thing — such a wish is masochistic. Yes, I long for a world that won't easily fly apart, but, thank God, I also like it that the world is like a birthday party. But I regularly come back to Science and Reason, the instruments that I think will keep me safe and on track, safe from my other addictions: irony and vulgarity. Sensible people work hard, do their duty, and make their mark, don't they?

But my Science and Reason are corrupt: I use them against one another, to cast doubt on Science and Reason themselves, and to persuade myself I've found out something shocking, something more important than good sense and ordinary human decency. My revelation is that poets, playwrights, and novelists are the only psychologists who think seriously about human life, who haven't abandoned the ship.

These artists haven't nailed down the cause of craziness and worry any more than psychiatrists; all too often, they try to convince us that madness is simple: it's caused by a broken heart. Although they're wrong, they've edged closer to truth than the psychiatrists who dream up chemicals and brain abnormalities. We all know that a broken heart — note the metaphor — drives us mad, murders sleep, and sears the nerves. Although I argue for the wisdom of novelists and poets, I split-think like everyone else. I confess I still want to convince myself, though it's a misplaced aim, that scientists, the people who celebrate reason, are always best at ferreting out the truth.

Reason and intellect are handy for other things, too. Having learned the art of argument from my quarrelsome mother, I'm helped by them to outwit people with whom I disagree. My arguing is designed to convince me I'm not my mother; at the least, I don't argue like her. Were I she I'd be a sissy and a blamer, but since my arguments are rational, her habit of blaming obviously — *obviously* — doesn't apply to me.

Secretly, it lets me *be* my mother, but in so disguised a form I don't know it. I tell myself that my interest in the arts doesn't mean I'm a sissy; it's just that intellect and reason have led me to conclude that such interests are the finger-kissing ultimate in intellectuality. It's my own discovery of the sublime, I guess, placebo-like in its power to soothe my soul.

This fragment of self-analysis is science, or so many psychoanalysts argue. I did, too, for many years. But others think it's navel-gazing hokum. What if, instead, it's just this era's fashion to think it creative and inventive to examine who we are. The heroic belief that a sublime development of myself is possible is Romanticism, an idea thousands of years old: Ovid's *Metamorphoses* is the prototypical catalogue of transformative change.

I'm not illustrating the cure by Reason and Logic by telling the story of a patient; I'm suggesting that I'm as good a case study as any other. Therefore think of what follows as me in action. Take the arguments seriously, but keep in mind that my conclusions aren't conclusive. It is just as important to observe the back-and-forth movement of my mind, my tendency to befuddle myself with Reason (wasn't there a god or goddess called *Loge*?). My logic doesn't sail me across the seven seas, it sails me towards beliefs I had embraced long before I drew up anchor, set my sails, and got logical about it. I am, of course, another merry crewmember on the Ship of Fools.

As the ancient Greeks said, celebrating logic is my *átã*, my faith or divine infatuation, the way I keep my psychological balance. I earn my passage on the Ship of Fools by sometimes going too far, getting too clever, challenging conventional thinking too much.

As I immerse myself in Science and Reason (I'm being coy; I'm really going to wage intellectual warfare), I'll cut back on making observations about myself and leave that to you. The things that come into focus about me should be treated as primary data, and you should study them on your own. You'll notice that I often confess my folly; that's an observation you'll use when you put together your portrait, a datum in your psychiatric observations. You should also notice I'm doing a lot of coaching and charming. Work that into your case study.

Instead of keeping me on the straight and narrow, a sensible good citizen, logic is my way of being nuts, crazy, a psychiatric madman; the rhetorical flourishes that I throw in aim to jolly you along as I make my arguments, but they also give away my inner corruption. Isn't something going wrong when a logician-scientist flirts with literary gestures and dramatic metaphors? The fact that this style cures my soul neither makes it a disease, a criterion for disqualification from the human race, nor does it mean I need treatment. It's just me. This is a case history, an illustration of the ceremonial way of life that is my own placebo cure, shared by lots of others with intellectual pretensions.

By claiming to know the truth, priests destroy human perfection. In other words, every truth claim shrinks the kaleidoscope of life and limits free imagination. Modern priests come in two versions: the Believers and the Skeptics. Both use reason to convince themselves they've found the answer. I weep in despair at the virtually identical reasonable arguments of Palestinians and Israelis, each side certain that reason proves it right. Believers possessed by the goddess "Ardour" (I just invented her), whose divine infatuation is Palestinian or Israeli, can't be talked to.

Believers claim they discover solid facts. Uncompromising scientists and fundamentalist clergymen are the obvious examples, sure that they know scientific and spiritual truths. Believers inspire us because, with answers — *especially* with answers — and a bit of charisma, they excite us into signing on.

The second group, Skeptics, claim reason leads in the opposite direction: nothing can be known and nothing discovered. Facts are only current thought, practical for one purpose or another, but never a final answer. Skeptics tend to be philosophers, linguists, and scientists interested in theory and the philosophy of science. Their heroes? Nietzsche and Wittgenstein, darkly obscure and theoretical.

Skeptics, on the surface, aren't inspiring; they are spoilsports, wet blankets, deadbeats, and just plain no fun. They carry no banners aloft for us to cheer. On the other hand, there are cults galore of deconstructionists, Derrida-ists and Wittgenstein-ists. Communal hysteria is for those who believe in Scientology, those convinced being reborn in Christ is the final answer, *and* for those convinced that disabling everyone else's beliefs leads to salvation. Reason has derailed them all.

Believers and Skeptics are religious. They are enchanted by the sublime, something transcendent, as long as it's *their* sublime — a demonstration of the fact that its real purpose is to give them comfort. Metaphorically their souls are healed by the transcendent truths towards which they've journeyed. If they heal themselves by finding a truth to believe in, it's the kind of ceremonial self-treatment I call a placebo. To say Believers and Skeptics are administering a placebo cure to themselves is surely true, but they would only reluctantly agree; placebos, they would insist, are for treating symptoms, especially the symptoms of silly people who complain too much. The word "ceremony" wouldn't suit them any better, yet all cling to their own comforting ceremonial beliefs and rituals, each precious and self-defining.

It's a waste of time being annoyed when Believers and Skeptics peddle their wares. Even yelling "You're superstitious fools" is a waste of breath. If we must judge, best to concentrate on the people themselves and judge them only on how they live: the guys who believe in tangible reality are heroes, adulterers, and crooks just as often as the doubters who believe in nothing.

Because they believe, psychiatrists who belong to the first group throw up diagnostic disease categories, medical-psychiatric disorders. For these, they have no evidence. Thirty years ago, they were called functional or idiopathic disorders (from the Greek word *idios*, "unique"), an acknowledgement that we didn't know what was going on. Now, fibromyalgia, all psychiatric disorders, chronic fatigue syndrome, and many more are passionately believed in, both by certain doctors and by advocacy groups, all unaccountably hysterical on behalf of their disorders. What in the world is there to get hysterical about? Why is it a moral issue if we do or don't know whether something exists?

I once audited a practitioner under scrutiny by his professional college. Every patient — I inspected two hundred charts — carried the diagnosis of chronic fatigue syndrome. He had carefully recorded in his notes his patients' day-to-day activities, and his typical responses to what they told him: "You shouldn't have done that; you should have gone home and rested."

Another practitioner, who also conscientiously recorded the questions he asked his patients, found evidence of childhood sexual abuse in all his patients. He pressed them to remember the abuse, sometimes employing a trick Freud had used early in his career. He told his patients to close their eyes, and that he would place his hand on their foreheads. Then he told them, at the instant of his touching, they would remember the abuse. He also had a high index of suspicion that his patients might have multiple personality disorder. He asked them about it, but not as urgently as he demanded that they remember being abused.

I confess I'm a skeptic. We're valuable because we keep the world thinking, which is handy when frantic believers try to sell a bill of goods about unknown or imaginary illnesses. My opposite-minded colleagues, those dedicated to discovering facts, are just as valuable;

they discover medical diseases and biologically effective treatments (though not in psychiatry). That's why they are medical diagnosticians and surgeons and I'm a psychiatrist.

When diseases are treated, there's a tendency to self-correction. Treatments that work eventually trump treatments that have only ceremonial effects. Untreatable diseases like terminal cancer are also candidates for placebos because nothing can trump them; we have nothing curative for terminal cancer patients. Medical doctors rarely worry about ceremonial treatments for incurable patients because, just as in psychiatry, placebo treatments for them always spring up, only to go out of fashion in a few months or years. These placebos are a problem only when people squander their savings on them.

I'm a medical doctor, well trained in scientific rationality, and have all the standard, automatic reactions to those who "fall for" placebo cures. *They're superstitious fools* is what I want to say. It takes effort, painful effort, to smarten up about this, because tolerance comes to me only after hard work, accompanied by plenty of inner wailing and gnashing of teeth; I have to struggle against my own will. Neither my scientific reactions nor my tolerant reactions are based on reason; they are, as Søren Kierkegaard taught us, leaps of faith. Kierkegaard himself may have had more exalted notions of what constitutes a leap of faith, but I'm damned if I can see how faith in religion differs from faith in reason. Scientists may be insulted when I say their approach is only one of many faith positions, but it is. My faith position, the one I've adopted only with difficulty, is to say that those who use placebos are participants in important cultural ceremonies.

Again and again, we're tempted to think we've got an answer. Only a moment ago, this "answer" flitted through my mind: "Maybe institutionalizing critique will prevent trouble. When we've reasoned something out, there ought to be a rule that the conclusion has to be bombarded by other opinions, pitted against heart and guts, emotions consulted, plus spontaneity, impulsivity, instinct. Then we'd be safe from conclusions derived only from reason.

"When we passionately believe something is true and right, believe it in our hearts, in other words, we should change gears, approach the issue with reason, subject it to rational critique, tests, and experiments. Every alternative ought to be brought into play before opinion is accepted."

Trusting in the clash of two inclinations may be better than trusting the supremacy of one, but every answer, including my critique answer, leads to more muddle. A formulaic reason-versus-the-gut style of life doesn't immunize us against folly any better than anything else: reason versus humanity; skepticism critiqued by tradition; humanity subjected to common sense. Critique is important and neglected but, elevated to ideology, leads only to more wheel spinning. Unfortunately for rationalists like me, subversive poets like W. H. Auden remind us that, as the title of one of his poems says, sometimes it's better to "Leap Before You Look." Life is fabulous, also disorderly and unsatisfying.

.+.+.+.

Despite the hoopla about brain diseases, even the strangest of behaviours are mysterious. Whether we say such people have mental disorders, or call them "nuts," "crazy," or "neurotic," there are only two ways to react. First, if the person is personally at peace, dangerous neither to himself nor others, we must pull back, not talk of sickness, and say, simply, "That's the way he's come to live." This response is simple but rare; most of us are judgemental and intolerant, not inclined to react this way. Instinctively, reflexively, automatically, we react diagnostically, and want to get straight what others are up to. It's hard to stand by when unconventionality is extreme and socially disapproved — such as living as a derelict, hallucinating, or embracing a weird religion — especially if it involves someone we love.

Intolerance of oddity is a modern habit, rationalized as medical or human concern. It's a fashion, our current style of thinking, of which psychiatrists are the anointed spokesmen. This fashion is unacceptable, our era's prejudice, and when we indulge in it, we've become racist clones. Unfortunately, as with all cultural conventions, we are blind to it, convinced we are doing the right thing.

The second reaction to "mental disorders" should come into play only if the person himself wants help. If he does, he'll go to a doctor, who will acknowledge that the dilemma is understandable and fits with what happens to others. Doctors, if doing their job, will speak in medical language, which is exactly what the person needs: "You need to get into psychotherapy (take this drug; come into the hospital)."

What such doctors are saying — their deep message — is different. They are actually saying, "Here's the proof you will be okay." If the doctor is a psychotherapist he or she will continue, "I have a ritual I perform. It's called psychotherapy, and it's been around long enough that we've gotten most of the kinks out of it. I'm properly trained and usually immune to slipping into trite slogans and useless advice. Since we're going to work together psychotherapeutically, you can assume it's clear that what you're going through is well known, and a way of comforting you is available."

Agreeable ceremonial treatments are superb therapeutic instruments, and psychotherapy and drug treatments are the ones most commonly offered, not because they cure, but because they are our culture's current craze, our *átã*, or "divine infatuation." I'm all in favour of wisdom-informed brands of psychotherapy and drug treatment; I'm dead against naive abuse of both these methods. I don't know how to drive myself and the rest of the world into the arms of the goddess Wisdom (the culture of ancient Greece celebrated conventional gender rules and therefore insisted that *mêtis*, divine intelligence, can only be got from a woman) and get her to show us how to do the hard work of being good psychiatrists.

Why do I call on an ancient goddess for help? Because a lot of psychotherapy is practised badly, an easy habit to fall into if, no matter what we do, most patients get better. The same goes for drug treatments that, to my horror, are often used to shut people up or get rid of them. Discriminating use of neuroleptics and lithium may be helpful, although antidepressants, because the placebo response to them is so powerful, don't inspire confidence. Using drugs wisely means using them less often than we now do. If we get the fix I've asked for — *mêtis* from Pallas Athena — we might even invent new ceremonies.

But ceremonies aren't easy to design; having a mind of their own, they take it upon themselves to spring up spontaneously. Cultural tastes are like some invisible beast whose behaviour can be neither predicted nor fathomed, their unpredictability puzzling and unexplainable. Perhaps that's why philosophers have so often invented world spirits or historical inevitabilities — anything, as long as it helps them to explain. We're all detectives and theorists, recklessly inventing answers, as though it's unbearable there are things we don't know.

It's okay to talk about people being sick or unwell, but if it's decided — and this is what's going on nowadays — that unconventional behaviour is a disease, there's no choice: we have to do something medical and believe it's curing something. If we're moralists and view such actions and reactions as a sin or crime, there's also no choice: we've got to make a negative judgement, apply a penalty, or both.

Our species seems bound to make judgements. Early in my career, hydrotherapy (immersion in tubs of circulating water), wet packs (wrapping patients in wet sheets), and dry packs were frequent psychiatric treatments, designed to soothe and relax. But soon I noticed they were also punishments: "If you don't settle down, we'll have to put you in a pack." And sure enough, the ceremony of putting someone in a pack became a punitive, prison-guard procedure: burly attendants would corner the miscreant (who, moments before, had been "sick") and forcibly carry him to bath or bed for the compulsory application of water or sheets. I remember watching in amazement as patients were tossed back and forth as attendants mummified the patient in their sheet-pack, an institutionalized version of being enveloped in Saran Wrap, like spiders skilfully wrapping their prey in silk.

Now that we're modern and scientific, are things different? Of course not. There's no longer the threat of a pack; we have our own procedures: "If you don't settle down we're going to have to sedate you," and "If you don't come in to the hospital on your own we're going to have to certify you." There's no escaping moral judgements, which are barely disguised as medical diagnoses and treatments. We deeply dislike people who act oddly or crazily; we're determined to confine and subdue them, and, when they are dangerous, so we should. But why not speak plainly rather than using euphemisms like "treatment"?

The oft-cited miracle of neuroleptic drugs is less a miracle than is commonly thought; psychiatric wards weren't much different when I was a medical student in 1955 than they are now. Then, I witnessed a one-time schoolmate who was permanently in a sheet pack, flushed with fury, with bulging purple veins on throat and forehead, neck tendons taut. A few years later he was quiet, but apathetic and disfigured by serious drug side effects. I can't say one state is better than the other.

+ + +

Were we able to convince psychiatrists that odd and unacceptable behaviour — and all the other troubles of life — is unending, we'd have a chance of getting them to give up the disease idea, the disease idea that is a euphemism for bad, awful, unacceptable behaviour. Since there's currently no serious debate, especially in academic departments of psychiatry, we'll have to endure the current state of affairs for quite a while.

The scientific bias of medicine ought to nag clinical psychiatrists enough to get them thinking, but there's no sign this will happen. Success as an academic depends on flogging the disease (biologically inferior, bad, unacceptable) model. The research industry requires this, as it absorbs money, largely from taxpayers and from sick people who have to buy its drugs. I'm only reassured when I talk to real scientists, those who, rather than being caught in the frantic search for another bacterium, chemical, or lesion that might cause something, just do their basic research.

Thinking seriously means thinking about ourselves. This grueling practice hurts like the devil. Although lots of us like some of the things that hurt — chopping wood, jogging, and sacrificing ourselves for those we love — few people like the interior struggle required to rethink our most basic assumptions. We're stuck with the status quo, pious assertions of concern about non-existent diseases and their treatments. There are scientific meetings, but instead of debate, psychiatrists do a chant, no different from the repetitive chants I heard when I visited an

Indian ashram: recitals of what the debaters already believe in. I want to say that crazy illusions will fade, but history suggests I'm wrong.

The belief that psychiatric patients have biological abnormalities limits thinking, if not bringing it to a stop; if genes and chemistry are it, what else is there to think about? Those who think this are mixing up materialism with science; they conclude that, if they can focus on humans as physiologically living stuff, this makes them scientists. This logical blunder isn't hard to figure out. Materialism isn't science; it's a philosophical view of the world. That view can, of course, be tackled scientifically, and it has been, with spectacular success, in all branches of medicine except psychiatry. In my specialty, no material abnormalities have ever been found. Yet modern psychiatrists keep insisting there are material causes for psychiatric disorders, which illustrates that they speak for a faith position, an ideology, certainly not for science.

Oftener than not, our patients tell us they are better, exactly what we want to hear. Our empirical traditions make us vulnerable; empiricism suggests that, if it works, we are on the right track. But that's a far cry from knowing a disease has been cured. Any doctor can subdue symptoms, of course, but that has nothing to do with either disease or materialism. Whisky cures my nervousness every time — but I have no disease. A scientific approach evades this error; Koch's postulates, taught to all medical students, require us to find objective abnormalities that are modified by our treatment. If there are no objective findings, and no objective changes following treatment, there is no disease. These postulates — rules — immunize us against thinking that, because our patient says he's better, something has been cured.

Once we know there are no physical findings, we ought to know what to do: conduct ourselves professionally; offer medical counsel; do this knowing it is a medical ritual; expect the unhappy person to be comforted and to have gained courage. If we are trained as psychotherapists, our management can be more ambitious: symbolic understanding of the meaning of symptoms. Blindness to ceremonial obligations makes it impossible to have serious discussions about which ceremonies might be best, and I'm not suggesting we invent new ones. I'm talking about intellectual ferment: a debate that pits drugs, trivial psychotherapies, and in-depth psychotherapies against one another.

I'm claiming for psychiatry — and for general medicine — enormous territory. If we play a central role in the culture, psychiatry's job is bigger and harder than we've thought. We humans are hardwired to skilfully negotiate the networks of symbols, rules, roles, and customs that we ourselves have invented. Psychiatrists, key players in this buzzing, electro-social field, must be careful, think hard about the methods we have on sale. If we know the rules, customs, ideas, and symbolic roles worth hanging on to, we'll be positioned to inspire our culture. If, for example, psychiatry judges some citizens to be biologically inferior, the culture, because it respects our opinions, will accommodate itself, even to this evil idea. If we stand *against* judging some citizens as inferior, the culture will accommodate *that* idea. Much more is at stake than "disease" and "treatment."

Although many, especially psychiatrists, have trouble with these ideas, lots of people tackle this topic successfully. I recently talked to a member of a self-help organization called the "Recovery Movement." To my surprise, she thought about unhappiness and madness exactly as I do, so I asked if the word "recovery" didn't contradict her point of view. She herself knew the word was problematic, and reported that this had been the topic of a long discussion at one of her organization's meetings. Later, she referred to herself as a "psychiatric survivor." I smiled. Before I could tease her by saying, "Survivor?" she smiled herself.

✧ ✧ ✧

An analogous faith in biology characterized nineteenth-century psychiatry, but between then and now, Freud's psychology dominated for eighty years. The intervening period wasn't just the psychology of Freud; he was part of a late-nineteenth-century interest in hysteria, dissociative states, railroad spine, multiple personalities — the nineteenth-century equivalents of chronic fatigue, attention deficit, and fibromyalgia. Psychiatrists explained these conditions by postulating "dissociated psychical contents," their term for the unconscious.

Freud, by being persuasive and literary (he once won the Goethe prize for literature), popularized the unconscious and promoted serious speculation about the deeper workings of the mind. Mental disorders aren't caused by bad chemistry, said Freud; it's a pathogenic secret that's causing the trouble.

The pathogenic-secret idea was also misleading. Before this, abnormalities of the brain had to be compensated for; under Freud the pathogenic secret had to be cleaned out. It doesn't matter that Freud gave up that theory; this was the idea that stuck in people's minds. Freud's later thinking was more sophisticated and what he'd once called psychological illness became a variant on ordinary folly, the outcome of each person's unexpected forms of psychological ingenuity.

The idea that madness and common folly are on a continuum was intolerable to both psychiatrists and the public; labelling oddity as disease or as sin seems to be automatic. In the long run, the idea that there is no essential difference between madness and normality — that people differ only qualitatively — was fatal to psychological psychiatry. Once it sank in that Freud was arguing that there is no dirty pathology to be cleaned out of people's minds, psychiatry retreated from psychoanalysis. Its revolutionary nature was too much to swallow.

Two different psychiatric streams developed. The first abandoned psychology completely and became modern psychiatry's mainstream, those who retreated to thinking of patients as biologically crippled. The second stream, the weakened Freudian schools, were equally troubled by Freud's liberalism — his acceptance of unusual behaviour as variant rather than illness — and urgently conjured up more and more theories of *mental* pathology. What patients did was no longer an angle on ordinary conduct, and certainly not something we all have in common.

The idea of the pathogenic secret has good credentials. It's the stuff of myths: hysterically dramatic, a caricature of real life, and comforting because of its simple, black-and-white character. It takes us straight to the Garden of Eden and the secrets of the Tree of Knowledge. Fascinated by secrets, we're never finished trying to find the "true" nature of things in general and of mental suffering in particular. The myths — Nietzsche and Schopenhauer get a share of the honour for this — teach us to ally ourselves to the uncovering attitude that, most of all, lives on in literature, theatre, and film. But it's barely breathing in psychiatry.

Not knowing is good for us. We're interesting as a species precisely because, if not trapped in convention, we invent and reinvent the world, create narratives about what's going on. Even well-known stories get reworked; there's no end to versions of *Hamlet* and *The Sopranos*. When we think we've got the *real* story, biology for example, we risk saying, "Ah ha, I've got it. Now that we've got the answer, Utopia is in sight." Utopians invariably depend on the idea that the universe is tidy and follows laws that, if properly applied, will perfect the world. When applied to human actions, I say, induction, deduction, the laws of the excluded middle and of sufficient cause, even reason itself, are curses. Platonic rationalists are as much a menace as those who, equally starry-eyed, believe in transcendental experiences. All utopians flirt with genetic purification and engineering. Think Hitler, the Inquisition, and Sadaam, all salesmen for simple answers.

A "sane" world is dangerous, limited and narrow-minded, reductionistic and lacking complexity, a world so hell-bent on sanity that, whenever a rational social order has to come to pass (under the Khmer Rouge, in Stalin's Soviet Union, in Maoist China), citizens, if they want to survive, must pretend to be rational robots: no mystery, silliness, or unconventionality allowed. It's the danger of the Brave New World that makes cultures throw up odd, dissident thinkers, who, by stirring up change, help us sidestep the tendency to hope for a final answer.

It's stupid to ask psychiatrists to make people behave — work hard, get married, make babies, be successful, dress nicely — and even more stupid for a psychiatrist to agree. Not surprisingly, even psychiatrists like me — those who see our job as subversive — secretly hope our patients will behave. As Nietzsche taught us, cultural conventions are demanding: "Prohibitions, cruel prohibitions, are what characterize a culture and make it work."

✢ ✢ ✢

Hamlet and Anna Karenina found themselves in one-dimensional psychological traps they couldn't get out of, stuck without new ways to understand dilemma. Suicide is a trap, self-devised, thinking there's only one way out. But deciding that suicide must, at all costs, be prevented is a complementary trap. Our first and most automatic reaction is to try to stop someone from killing himself, but it's not so simple: for some, self-slaughter is the answer. For others it's being a homemaker or a biker, earning entry to a madhouse, or becoming a professor of theoretical physics.

CHAPTER ELEVEN

BEAUTY, TASTE, THE ARTS

I'VE SPENT MY LIFE ATTEMPTING TO BE normal, working hard, earning money, making friends, and remembering birthdays. But in May 2004, I forgot the birthdays of Mariah and Alex, two of my grandchildren, and of Diana and Paul, two of my children. If four important birthdays occur in one month they're hard to forget, and the truth is they hadn't completely slipped my mind. Without signs of Alzheimer's, I can't be let off the hook. I'd *neglected* the birthdays, failed to attend and focus.

I know what was going on: I was writing this book. In a way, I *wanted* to be negligent, enacting a stereotype that includes not shaving regularly, dropping clothes to the floor, and not phoning friends: I'm an artist wannabe.

Real artists (despite pretensions, psychiatrists are only half-artists, and only in their consulting rooms) transform the world into art. When they make love, they watch. They don't merely beat wives or hire rentboys to strike them with cats-o'-nine-tails, nor do they merely write books or direct plays. They watch: "I am a camera," said Christopher Isherwood.

Above the oracle at Delphi is inscribed *Gnothi se auton*, usually translated as "Know thyself." But Socrates says there's a better translation: "Look at thyself." The command demands we should be artists of self-watching. Psychiatry's job is to encourage this style of thinking.

Each artist watches in his own way, just as I, half-artist, study patients my own way. In the consulting room, I'm lost in thought, watching from a non-existent vantage point, baffled and fascinated. I'm a pondering fool, a fanatic of observation and sparse comment.

Pondering fool that I am, should my patient comment on the weather, I narrow my eyes and think. A cheerful greeting, acknowledgement of a new wound on my face, or praise of a painting on my wall, garners only more of my pondering madness. And should the patient tell me to get fucked, fire me, or spread malicious rumours, I don't shift ground. I'm half-mad with pondering. When with my patient, I forget all birthdays, decline all realities, and insist (without saying so) that what transpires on my couch is, exclusively and brilliantly, artistic narrative and performance. By making only an artistic critique, I drive my patients crazy, the craziness that is the cure, the transformation of themselves into works of art.

Skilled psychiatrists don't judge; they view what patients say and do as neither good nor bad, nor as normal (whatever that might be) or pathological. Instead, psychiatrists insist on finding interest and, note that everything can be aestheticized; babies, derelicts, my smelly seatmate on the subway in today's heat wave — even pus and blood, piss and shit — can be subordinated to the artistic eye. But it's hard. It demands that the psychiatrist be in a state of fascination, a state of mind hard to achieve through the will. I'm tempted to say that, because fascination can't be done on purpose, psychiatrists are born, not made. But generalizations aren't a good idea.

Like everyone, psychiatrists are in the habit of deciding things are good or bad, right or wrong. To transform the world — and patients — into works of art is possible only when psychiatrists wrench themselves into an odd observational stance, sometimes easily, sometimes only with effort. Yet it's the demand good psychiatrists make upon themselves.

Despite pretensions, I'm only a half-artist, embedded as well in the real world; were I not, I couldn't make a living. My artistic observations are played off against reality. In blocks of forty-five minutes, I sell my time for hard money. If patients don't attend, stand on their heads, or read magazines, it is performance art. If they don't pay, it's performance art, too, but in this instance — and it's the only one — financial realities outrank theatre; the contract is terminated. Although I'm a hard-headed half-artist, I'm also a hard-headed half-businessman.

If, having undergone the ceremonial treatment, patients join in and becomes artistic observers of their own ways, they will have effected a cure of the highest quality. Having learned in parallel to me, who, for weeks or months, will have pondered their many performances on my consulting-room stage, patients will have achieved aesthetic healing. Stingy with words, I will have given them reviews of what I've seen; once they've become my aesthetic comrades and critics of their own speeches and behaviour, patients will proceed alone. They will have been cured.

You will have noticed that I'm fond of the cure by aestheticism.

❖ ❖ ❖

In 2001, at the *Staatsoper* in Berlin, I attended a performance of Leoš Janáček's opera *The Cunning Little Vixen*. Berliners consider this a children's opera so, all dressed up, there were many boys and girls excitedly anticipating what was to come. Abandoning artistic pretensions (jeans, failure to bathe), I adapted to Berlin formality and wore a dark suit and sober tie.

I loved *The Cunning Little Vixen*, thrilled by the music, singing, acting, staging — everything. It begins in a forest, humming with life and colour — flowers are blooming, insects buzzing, animals playing and hiding. But I noticed something else: the opera was raunchy. It's spring, and the main character, a young vixen, spends plenty of time prancing around nude, not even a bit of gauze to cover her crotch. The rooster on a nearby farm, the sweet hornet Eros stinging him, diligently humps his harem of hens. "My God," I said to myself. "What will the children think?"

I spied on the children near me, but none betrayed uneasiness; there wasn't a giggle to be heard. I wasn't surprised at the nudity — German stages are notorious for nudity and the bizarre — nor was I surprised at the calm demeanour of the children in the audience. Children know more than we think. But like a half-artist, I noticed.

I was strongly affected by the opera and rode the U-Bahn to my hotel in a daze. *The Cunning Little Vixen* had cured my cynicism about the stupidity of bureaucracy: someone had put this artistic feast together. Janáček had written the score, musicians had played the music, and performers had sung and acted. Designers, directors, lighting experts, stage hands, and an advertising department had worked together, along with the architects and builders of the opera house, politicians that raised the money, and a music director, Daniel Barenboim, who had planned the season and conducted the orchestra.

My cynicism had vanished, but an extra glow had been added. The world became glorious and fine; even the dilapidated U-Bahn subway cars looked tidier. I'd become more tolerant. "Who am I to judge?" I thought.

All placebo cures, including the cure by aestheticism, are versatile: as often as not, their opposite works just as well. Fasting is a terrific cure, but so is feasting. And just as "highbrow" aestheticism is an excellent placebo cure for some, "lowbrow" aestheticism cures plenty of others. No one knows which is which: is it the opera or popular music that's genuine? Should psychiatry's music therapists play Bach or the Beastie Boys?

The glow I experienced after seeing *The Cunning Little Vixen* lasted for several weeks, and I anticipated Toronto's opera season more than ever. Usually preoccupied by too many realities, that night I'd been reminded of Peter Pan: "Don't forget to believe in fairies!" Aesthetic bliss, rare, hard to find, leads us to pause — to exist — for a moment. Once I had paused and regrouped, stupid politicians and administrators didn't look as stupid as before. Despite a thrilling performance of another of Janáček's operas, *Jenufa* in Toronto, a repeat cleansing of dark attitudes, the glow eventually faded. Cynicism returned: I'm writing this book, aren't I?

Were they real artists, psychiatrists, when in performance with their patients, still couldn't create aesthetic bliss. Unfortunately for both, the warts and pimples of each intrude. As they enter their patients' lives, psychiatrists unearth, alongside talents and beauty, stinks and stains — and they don't like it. For patients it's harder; because psychiatrists are quiet, their secret blemishes and bigotries take longer to figure out. But aesthetic bliss? Only momentarily. Like falling in love, getting a book published, or winning the lottery, the bliss is temporary. Captain Ahab's toast to his crew in *Moby Dick* — straight rum — gets it right: "Like life, gulped and gone."

But the cure through aesthetics makes sense — a lot of sense. In films, books, and operas we discover human nature writ large, ourselves and our fellows portrayed in action, with complexities, blemishes, and perversities included. Like psychiatrists, art invites us to wrestle with ghosts. Clark Kent and Emma Bovary are both you and me, our sisters and brothers as well.

✢ ✢ ✢

The idea of being transformed — in my case from cynic to romantic — is a humanity-defining perception of life, and the foundation of all notions of cure and change: a rebirth fantasy. That's why Ovid wrote the *Metamorphoses*, and why his tales are made into movies. A modern example is Bill Gates, a classic version of the revenge of the nerd; three thousand years earlier, Achilles (I guess he was a sissy) erupted into battle mode when Patroclus, his boyfriend, was killed. Whether it's a cripple transformed into superhero, Peter Parker turning into Spiderman, or the mild-mannered Bruce Banner bursting out of his clothes to become the Hulk, transformation stories are everywhere: the Frog Prince, Snow White, satisfaction after a long bike ride, hopes for my next patient. Every one of these stories is serious. When, at the end of *Spiderman 2*, Peter Parker decided he'd go back to being a superhero — reborn — I got tears in my eyes.

In recognition of this truth, *The Cunning Little Vixen* is about metamorphosis and rebirth. The little vixen grows up, finds a foxy boyfriend, and bears a litter of pups. Tragically, she is shot by a hunter. But the opera ends as it began: a forest, birds, bugs, flowers, playful young foxes. It's spring. Life has begun again.

Does this mean that ceremonial cures — the effect on my outlook that I've just described — are fakes, flash-in-the-pan trickery? Not at all. I say that this, like all well-matured events that embed us in our culture, is a permanent and substantial cure: it has added wisdom to my repertoire. I may be a cynic forever, but I also know better, and am liable to think twice. Knee-jerk scoffing and scorning won't ever again be so easy.

❖ ❖ ❖

In 2002, an editorial in the *British Medical Journal*[1] suggested we should "spend (slightly) less on health and more on the arts." Health, the editorialist argues, would probably be improved.

> The first problem with advancing such an unpopular argu-
> ment is to define health. It must be more than "the absence
> of disease," despite that being the working definition used
> by misnamed health services. Such a definition is inade-
> quate not only because of its narrowness and negativity but
> also because "disease" itself is so hard to define. The World
> Health Organization's definition of health as complete
> physical, mental, and social wellbeing understandably
> causes raised eyebrows. Human health can [have] nothing
> to do with perfection. Humans are highly imperfect crea-
> tures. But the WHO definition does acknowledge that there
> is more to health than physical completeness and an
> absence of pain. Indeed, the physical aspects of health may
> be the least important. Is it possible to be severely disabled,
> in pain, close to death, and in some sense "healthy"? I
> believe it is. Health has to do with adaptation and accept-
> ance. We will all be sick, suffer loss and hurt, and die.
> Health is not to do with avoiding these givens but with

accepting them, even making sense of them. The central task of life, believed people in medieval times, is to prepare for death.

✦ ✦ ✦

Among the sights of Mandalay, in Burma, is a gold *paya*. My guide, Than, was at pains to explain that the religious monuments are coated with real gold and the rainwater runoff is collected, because gold is washed off. The gold is then reclaimed from the wash water. Because he knew I was interested in healing, he showed me something else, a subsidiary shrine with a special Buddha. "This Buddha is for women who have difficulty in childbirth."

The story he told is mythology — literature — an artistic portrayal of a serious medical issue, its artistic rendering giving comfort to the troubled. I wrote the story down a few hours later.

A student once fell in love with his professor's daughter. He spoke to the professor and asked for her hand in marriage. The teacher told him he could marry his daughter if he collected for him one thousand fingers. The student was appalled and said no, but then his love got the better of him and he agreed.

He cut off many fingers and hung them around his neck. People feared him and moved away for safety, so there were no more people whose fingers he could collect. By then, he had 999 fingers hanging around his neck and needed only one more. He decided that, if he wanted to succeed in winning his bride, he'd have to get the last finger from his own mother.

Buddha intervened. "Instead of cutting off your mother's finger, we will have a competition," he said. "I will run and you must catch me." Unfortunately for him, the student could not catch Buddha, and eventually gave up the chase.

He also gave up his quest for fingers and for marriage. The fingers around his neck turned into finger-flowers, and he pursued a life of meditation and peace.

The people of the village came back and beat him, but he was tranquil because he had achieved Nirvana. Therefore, men with pregnant wives go to this shrine and pray their wives will have easy labours.

There's plenty of symbolism here, enough to tackle any sexual lesson that needs review; the story's bizarreness forces us to think. I have colleagues who also force themselves to think; they keep their minds in top condition by doing cryptic crossword puzzles every day. Others tune up by reading difficult books and poetry, or by listening to Tom Waits and Arnold Schoenberg. Going to movies and playing bridge also do the trick.

Vladimir Nabokov's *Pale Fire*[2] is, arguably, his greatest novel. I'm devoted to being an intellectual, so my irritation by the book, and lack of interest in it, makes me feel inferior. The book is a puzzle, and deciphering it is hard work. Were I a schoolboy, and a teacher assigned the book, I could probably decipher it as a work assignment, but there'd be no thrill, no sense of "divine infatuation." For some, puzzles like *Pale Fire* are thrilling — but not for me, a limitation I hate to admit. I say to my colleagues, *Don't worry so much about training yourself; remember to live.* It's advice I don't follow well.

✢ ✢ ✢

Doctors who give their patients a blue, sugar-filled gelatin capsule know they will likely achieve the same goal as the special Buddha. They can confidently say to their patients, "Jack, you're okay. I want you to take one of these before each meal for seven days. By then, you'll be feeling a lot better."

These doctors are speaking in code. What they mean is that Jack is out of sorts, disconnected from day-to-day life, an outcast so to speak. The medical message, translated into boring anthropological and psychological language, is this: "Jack, I'm one of the referees who supervise the struggles of life. You are temporarily down and out, but by coming, you've decided opera isn't the way you're inclined to cope with it today, nor is visiting a priest or a Buddhist shrine. 'Sickness' will be today's code word for your alienation. Don't worry, I'll shepherd you back where you belong. I don't count you as down and out, and suspect you're resilient. My job is to make symbolic statements and give pills laden with symbolic meaning. I don't make the sign of the cross or circumcise you, nor do I give a certificate of graduation or sing. But I'm important; I'm another of the guys who keeps you connected."

The doctor's words would carry more weight were she to administer the capsule to the patient herself, cautiously pick it up with tweezers, drop it into a glass of water, and say, "Wait until the fizzing stops and then drink it carefully." Drama makes the placebo (the bedside manner, the ritual) work better.

In Graham Greene's novel *A Burnt-out Case*,[3] Dr. Colin worries about the side effects of the drug he gives to a patient with leprosy:

> "It will be over soon," the doctor said. "You must be patient."
>
> . . . The D.D.S. tablets were not a simple cure. Reactions from the drug were sometimes terrible . . . in a few cases a kind of madness came over the mind in the hours of darkness. . . .
>
> The doctor said, "This will pass. One more night, that's all. Remember you have just to hold on. Can you read the time?"
>
> "Yes."
>
> "I will give you a clock that shines so that you can read it in the dark. The trouble will start at eight o'clock. At eleven o'clock you will feel worse. Don't struggle. If we tie your hands you will struggle. Just look at the clock. At one you will feel very bad, but then it will begin to pass. At three you will feel no worse than you do now, and after that less and less — the madness will go. Just look at the clock and remember what I say. Will you do that?"
>
> "My child . . ."

"Don't worry about your child. I will tell the sisters to look after him till the madness has gone. You must just watch the clock. As the hands move the madness will move too. And at five the clock will ring a bell. You can sleep then. Your madness will have gone. It won't come back."

A medical cure through pills and words is as important and valuable as an aesthetic vixen-cure. Each takes his cures where he finds them: attending the symphony; playing poker; writing letters to the editor; visiting a psychiatrist. Everything we do symbolizes our participation in the culture and our belief it will give comfort. Bizarre though his choice may seem, even a crook is solving the problem of being a human and connecting himself to the culture.

Giving a blue, sugar-filled gelatin capsule isn't my way of delivering help; I do my curing with psychiatric talk. Although I've heard that all psychiatrists are nuts, I'm perfectly legitimate, and many like my talking ways — but there are other ways. Many ways make for generosity of spirit, a generosity too subtle for any known morality. Those narrowed by thinking they know the answers — cure chemical diseases of the brain, unearth Oedipus complexes, unmask non-empathic mothers — corrupt the world.

CHAPTER TWELVE

RESHAPING THE SOUL

I'VE PITTED REASON AGAINST AESTHETICS: getting things right against getting things beautiful. If one is inclined to organize the world in those ways, either illusion has the power to ease our minds, create a cure of life's woes. Set up as a sublime truth, each serves as lifeline and guideline, anchor and harbour — or a trap. And yet, though reason and aesthetics are opposites, they aren't as different as we think. They are bound by magic.

If I'm a psychiatrist, I'm also a shaman, magician, priest. In keeping with shamanic status, I'm obliged to create in my office an atmosphere of mystery and secrecy. I don't enchant my patients by falling into a trance, nor do I foam at the mouth. A proper doctor, I perform my shamanic acts through the means appropriate to our culture. The mysterious rituals of the psychiatrist are invisible to us, just as incense and wringing a chicken's neck are "invisible" to those accustomed to them as part of shamanic practices elsewhere.

Whether accomplished through drugs, shocks, or talk, the mysterious "presence" of the doctor transforms things. Don't get me wrong:

it's the doctor's duty to give symptomatic relief, a practice age-old and honourable. But it's not honourable if practitioners are convinced their patients' suffering is due to a disease and that they have cured something. Unhappily, probably because it smacks of magic, this psychological effect is in bad odour, so doctors think it's dishonourable to cash in on its spectacular effects. Our revulsion with spectacular cures, like those obtained at Lourdes or performed by faith healers on television, is caused by our own parochialism, bias, and intolerance in action.

My local car wash has a sign:

A CLEAN CAR LOOKS BETTER, DRIVES BETTER

Sure enough, when I drive away, the engine hums, the gears silently and smoothly change better than before. It's the placebo effect — working on me.

Herbs, foods, minerals, séances — and doctors — have the same good effect. The magical presence of the doctor is, and always has been, the doctor's most powerful medical weapon. It also confuses us, because we don't know whether our good results are due to the correction of a biological abnormality or to the wonderful suggestibility of patients, including our own when we are patients.

To the chagrin of many, the psychiatrist's talk offers — or ought to offer — a cure that differs radically from the usual kindness, encouragement, and sympathy, and from the usual and familiar pill placebos. What does the psychiatrist offer? An odd mixture: literature, humour, language, the horrible. Art bears a terrible insight for science, doctoring, and the medical tending of souls: the earnest pursuit of knowledge doesn't work well for psychiatrists. We're better off if we acknowledge ours as a poetic science, that our touchstones are lightness, magic, and wonder. How else could we know the weirdness and horror of real life?

Watching myself in action has little to do with science. I'm hung up on art, privilege it mercilessly, spilling the beans on my personal faith position, and offering clues to the suspicious about what might lie behind that public preoccupation.

✢ ✢ ✢

In what was once a church in San Juan Chamula, a Mayan village, a shaman was hard at work. She was exorcising a demon. More important, by urging her patient to co-operate with professional rituals, she was confirming his bond to his culture's conventions. As I watched, a musical analogy came to mind: this culture is mixed up. There's a dissonance here between Christianity and animism. The shaman helps the people to sound a resolving chord.

Centuries ago, the culture had been Christian, but in the 1930s, bandit-generals, psychopaths, and ideologues — especially ideologues — had banned the Roman Catholic Church. In remote parts of Chiapas, the Church has never recovered; in contrast, despite a similar animistic history, the voodooists of Haiti still consider themselves to be Catholics. By capitalizing on leftover bits of Roman Catholicism and animism, the latter supposedly long forgotten, the Mayan villagers have created a new religion. They believe in three realms: above is the realm of the gods; in the earthly realm live the Mayans; below the earth is the realm of the demonic. If it didn't antedate the three realms of Wagner's Ring cycle, this cosmos certainly parallels them: above the earth the gods; on the earth the giants; below the earth the Nibelungs. The Mayan gods include the many saints they've inherited from Christianity, plus the sun and Christ. All, I was told, are worshipped with equal reverence, often through the mediation of a major-domo, who is a religious official, but emphatically not a priest. There *are* priests, but they are excluded from all priestly functions except baptizing babies. Since dealings with the gods are in the hands of individual citizens or the major-domos, the priests are consigned to the periphery.

Shamans, on the other hand, deal with demons, the inhabitants of the nether realm, a task from which major-domos and priests are excluded. Shamans, intermediaries with the underworld, are the first to be approached at times of illness. I was told they are shrewd at distinguishing between physiological illness and visitations from the nether world, and, when necessary, refer patients to doctors. But I was also told their prestige is greater than that of medical doctors, because they have wider powers: they can remove evil influences from homes and crops.

I watched as one shaman — there were lots of them, all women — treated a painful arm. The ritual was spooky, sustained with smoke and awe-inspiring paraphernalia. She crouched on the floor of the church (was this still a church?) surrounded by the patient and her family. The shaman wore the same clothes as all the women in that community: a blue *rebozo* (a shawl or baby sling), or a gathered white blouse with embroidered trim, and a black wool wraparound skirt (the men wore baggy thigh-length trousers and black sarapes). Several times, she passed a chicken around the painful arm, then over a cluster of candles that she'd pasted to the floor, back and forth between the afflicted arm and the candles. I could smell singed feathers and feared for the chicken's eyes. But I needn't have worried; she suddenly wrung the chicken's neck and the treatment was over. A demon had been drawn from the painful wrist and transferred to the chicken. The chicken dead, the demon had been exorcised, and all was resolved. The tonic chord had been struck.

The shaman's patient had experienced one of the vital pleasures. Not lovemaking, music, career fulfillment, or playful fun, but nevertheless participation in a formal, traditional ceremony, in principle no different from vitamins and herbs given by a naturopath, placebo drugs prescribed by a family doctor, being blessed by a priest, or signing up for the talking rituals of a psychiatrist. The demand on the Mayan shaman corresponds exactly to the demand placed on Western doctors: give a service tailored to the culture.

These shamans are the front-line doctors and psychiatrists of the village culture. They deal with common, day-to-day ailments, the unwellness induced by the demonic world; this is the only service they dispense. In Western culture, psychiatrists are the people designated to deal with patients' demonic worlds, a role inherited from family doctors who gave it up when they became technologically sophisticated. The amazingly powerful turn to psychiatry and alternative medicine in recent years is a by-product of technological medicine and corresponds with the loss by family doctors of psychological skills and of important, mysterious elements in medical cures.

Twentieth-century psychiatrists — our society's shamans — act in accord with *our* culture's beliefs and values. Like the Mayans, we live in a medical culture caught between two sets of values: proudly sensible and scientific on the one hand; dispensing symbolic healing on the other. To this mix is added post-modernism: the twinkle in a good doctor's eyes gives away that he knows about skepticism and irony. Although we exploit the magical powers attributed to us, paradoxically, we also insist that doctors deserve no special prestige or authority. We do our job like anyone else.

Nowadays we throw up heroes cautiously. But our patients are old-fashioned, and insist on idealizing us. Instead of believing in the virtues patients confer on us, psychiatrists try to figure out what's going on. We analyze idealizations, not with a sledgehammer, but carefully, when the moment is ripe. It's hard to do; even though devoted to democratic and liberal attitudes, we like being admired. Worse than liking it is when we believe what's said.

✠ ✠ ✠

Irony and skepticism are neither angels and demons, born fully grown like Athena, nor are they aliens, previously unknown, who invade the modern world's soul. On the contrary; they've always been around. Socrates, St. Augustine, Shakespeare, and Goethe were well-known practitioners of the dark, ironic arts. The difference I'm trying to get at is that, in our era, irony and skepticism are central and constitutive. That's why we're "post-modern." I know being post-modern is kitschy, but it's much more; we ought now to recognize that belief is best held in abeyance. It's not that "anything goes" — although they may not fully own us, we all have standards — it's the important recognition that anything is worth reconsideration.

Our culture is far from uniform in its embrace of irony. Robert Hughes's *Culture of Complaint*[1] and Wendy Kaminer's *I'm Dysfunctional, You're Dysfunctional*[2] are strong critiques of ardent — and dangerous — beliefs that are rampant in our culture. The believers lampooned in these books are paired with corresponding placebo cures: for instance,

the 96 percent of us who supposedly come from dysfunctional families or have been victims of abuse, whether we remember it or not, are
cured by blaming someone.

I often wonder if my annoyance at the culture of victimhood is
misplaced, that people have always used that tactic to comfort themselves. But I suspect I'm partly right, that something common and
ordinary has got out of hand. Changing patterns of diagnosis reflect
the change.

When I was a young psychiatrist, post-traumatic stress disorder
didn't exist; we called it "compensation neurosis." Our diagnosis was
judgemental and invited us to get moralistic: "These patients are
fakers, out to get a payoff." The corresponding and currently favoured
diagnosis, post-traumatic stress disorder, is superficially empathic, but
leads into a different trap; it encourages us to think of our patients as
victims, an attitude that requires the patient to consider himself a
victim *of someone*. The risk is malignant blaming. Because they are preconceptions, both diagnostic labels are useless.

My day-to-day assumption is that psychiatric labels have little diagnostic and fewer therapeutic payoffs, so our patients need to be
thoroughly described — as good phenomenologists we're obliged to
do this *very* thoroughly — their histories examined and re-examined,
and intervention planned without a diagnosis.

⚜ ⚜ ⚜

I've gone on at length about my horror of belief. Does this mean that
I'm appalled at the practices of the Mayan shaman? And if not, what is
it that makes Mayan belief acceptable, although I write off alien possession as silly? The difference is that Mayan belief, by no means
perfect, has two essential qualities. First, it doesn't blame — it doesn't
advocate hatred and blaming — and, second, it's time-tested. The culture has had hundreds, perhaps thousands, of years to get the bugs out
of its system. That's why they've been able to keep on being Mayans
despite Christian impositions. The system is powerful because it
works, and it works because it's been painstakingly developed.

New Ageism, one of the cultures of complaint, blaming, and political correctness, is undeveloped, untested, and, most of all, has not been given due consideration. On the other hand, many generations of Mayans have pondered, discussed, and thought about how their system might best work. They've achieved this unwittingly, by a method of trial and error imposed on practices first chosen as a matter of taste. By virtue of time and thought, their system has cleansed itself — not perfectly, not forever, but just for now — of external scapegoating.

Currently, Mexico's Mayans haven't fallen for the easiest placebo cures, the one achieved by the external-devil trick. I'd like to say it is poorly trained practitioners who fall into this trap, but unfortunately it springs up everywhere: in hospitals, universities, opium dens, peacenik colonies. Medicine cabinets that shelve this rubbish, no matter where we find them, need regular cleanouts.

✦ ✦ ✦

None of the Ojibwa in Lansdowne House came to the nursing station on their own to see me, the visiting psychiatrist; Sally, the nurse who took me to their homes, identified all the patients. Psychiatry wasn't part of the culture. I felt like a fool, as though pretending I was a shaman in San Juan Chamula. I was being paid by the government to provide a service of little interest to the community. I was, in effect, a social policeman, and was taken to see people who made the nurse nervous. I thought the money ought to be paid to someone who would organize baseball games for the youngsters.

Only once did I feel like a psychiatrist. On the third morning I took a walk around the village; a ten-minute walk covered the whole length of the island. In a field, a young woman approached me, the only native who addressed me in the week I was there. I'd heard about this woman and her name, Agnes Yes-No, had stuck in my mind because she was a relative of Johnny Yes-No, a popular singer in Ontario (I'd not heard of him, but that's what I'd been told). She hemmed and hawed, and finally said she had a problem. Her complaint was strange: she was jealous of her husband. With some persuasion, she explained.

"All the men around here run around with women and wives are used to it. Nobody gets jealous because everybody does it."

"But jealousy is common," I said. "I'm not sure why this is a problem?"

"I know people get jealous in the south [Southern Ontario], because I seen it in movies."

"Movies?" I said.

"Yeah," she answered. "On Sunday nights, Father Ouimette [the priest] shows movies in the church. I seen the white women get jealous when their husbands go with other women."

"I still don't get why this bothers you?" I said.

Agnes Yes-No didn't have a quick answer. I could see she wanted to talk some more, but didn't know how to start.

"Well," she said, "it's the white women who get jealous. I'm like a white woman and not like an Indian. Maybe it's because my grandmother was white, so I'm jealous like a white woman."

It was my turn to think and stay quiet. Something was in my mind, but I didn't know whether I should say it. But as she lingered, I stuck my neck out. In all my years of practice, I'd never once addressed an adult patient by his or her first name, but, when I addressed Mrs. Yes-No, I couldn't use her title. Like all palefaces, I spoke to a native patronizingly, as though she were a child, and used her given name. But I gave her an adult message.

"Agnes," I said, "There's something else. Indians don't talk to psychiatrists. I've been coming here and to Port Hope for a couple of years, and you're the first person to come and tell me a problem. But white people go and talk to psychiatrists all the time. Maybe you talked to me because that's another way you feel like a white woman?"

"Yeah," she said. "I seen it in the movies."

✢ ✢ ✢

I was in Lansdowne House again the next year. Peter Lewin, a doctor from Toronto, was to go back to Sioux Lookout on the plane that had brought me in, but he and I had time to chat. "There's an old fellow with terminal cancer who's dying — Rick Boots. He'll probably die in the next twenty-four hours or so. There's nothing more to do, but you might want to pop in on him."

That afternoon, someone came to the nursing station to tell us Rick was dying, so I decided I should help out. When I walked outside and looked down the path, I could see many people standing outside Rick's house, more crowding the porch and doorway. I felt uneasy. In Toronto, I knew how doctors preside over a death, but in Lansdowne House I was unsure. Many thoughts rushed around in my mind. Once, I thought, priests presided over death, but we doctors have taken over. Although I assumed it was my job to take a central, reassuring, and comforting role in Rick Boots's death passage, I was still uncertain.

I pushed through the crowd and went into the house. No one gave me the welcome to which I was accustomed, "Oh, doctor, we're glad you're here." Instead, I was ignored. On the floor lay a man I assumed to be Rick Boots, propped up on heaps of blankets and pillows and cradled by two women, his sisters.

There was no need for me to be there. The family knew perfectly well how the death scene was to be managed. Rick was unconscious, and his sisters huddled on either side, wiping his face. To the side stood a lay brother, reading from a bible in the Ojibwa language. I was nothing more than an intruding freak, uncomfortable for having barged in on something private and sacred. I had no ceremonial role to play. The Ojibwa of Lansdowne House may have lost their cleansing rituals, but they hadn't lost their death rituals.

The next morning I heard that, at dawn, Rick's body had been taken by canoe to another island for burial. Not by motorboat, but by canoe, and accompanied by singing. Fortunately, I wasn't around to intrude into the family's privacy again.

These events illustrate no cure, unless we think presiding over life's crises — shepherding souls — is considered a cure. But it does illustrate that we have reassigned to medical doctors rituals that were once conducted by families and priests. We doctors don't think of these acts as rituals; to us, they are bureaucratic obligations and important guarantees that life-saving treatments haven't been given up on too soon. Since Rick Boots was beyond saving, perhaps in future such a death could be presided over by a government official, perhaps someone from the department of statistics.

�֍ �֍ �֍

If we doctors have taken it upon ourselves to preside over cultural rituals like death, we've done no harm. But if we shed other ritual responsibilities — understanding the psychology of our patients — we've neglected central elements in our work. If we don't see it when patients comfort themselves by the use of harmful psychological tricks (blaming others is the worst of these), we aren't doing our job. The danger posed by modern blamers is projection of their own villainy onto others. As Goethe said, "We are most offended by our faults when we discover them in others." The Mayan shamans blame demons, just as I — albeit with more conscious metaphoric intent — blame my patients' "demons" for their suffering. In contrast to the parent-blamers so common in North America, the assumptions of Mayan shamans aren't systematically persecutory.

The psychiatrists of whom I approve are unique only because they deliver our culture's message of liberal skepticism, the thing that makes the world mysterious and exciting. The fun of mystery and excitement is important, but not as important as something else: skepticism lets us change our minds. Their unwillingness to embrace any belief system makes my ideal psychiatrists the ideal carriers of another important cultural message: sidestepping fervent belief jigs the culture against tyranny.

Are there other analogies between my philosopher-psychiatrists and traditional shamans? Psychiatrists also believe their patients are possessed of a demon, but use a different name: transference re-enactment. Figures from the past are recognized in the patients' reactions to their doctors, reactions the psychiatrists do their best to figure out.

Does this exorcize the demons? Not exactly. It brings ancient presences to life, ghostly apparitions that, the more lively their presence in the psychiatrist's office, her ritual chamber, the more welcome they are. In contrast to those in Mexico, shamans like me are happy to have demons around, brought back to life. Once a demon becomes a presence, we're satisfied. Mayans differ in how they locate demons. For them, demons are underground or in the body; we psychiatrists vivify them in the imaginative mind.

✢✢✢

I'd not travelled until, after medical school, I went to Germany. The Second World War had been difficult; a few days after the war began, on a fine September morning in 1939, at 4:00 a.m., the Mounties arrived at our home in Lindsay, Ontario, and made off with my German father. He was held in secretly located camps for three years. The second hardship was that my secret, that I was "German," kept leaking out and then there'd be trouble with schoolmates. Don't get me wrong; my personal neurosis doesn't let me wail over such things. What matters is that the experience changed the shape of my soul, and eventually led me to go to Germany as soon as I finished my internship in 1958.

I was taken aback in the Köln (Cologne) railway station that people looked normal — rushing, lining up, eating, acting crabby. I realized I'd been expecting the German monsters I'd seen depicted in anti-German propaganda movies during the war when I was a child. This is a story I've told for forty years but recently, my urge to travel has taken on a new meaning. I no longer seem to be checking up on German monsters, I realize, but travel in order to check on whether Germans — and people that are suffering hardship — are okay. What strikes me now is that I consider them okay if people seem to fit in, are clear about their culture, the children good at their brand of play and mischief. And, of course, if young men and women are meeting.

This seems to be the case in most places I have travelled — except in the Sioux Lookout district in Northern Ontario. In the two communities I worked in, the Aboriginal culture looked wounded and the people unhappy. There seems to be no cultural nutrient for these Ojibwa, nothing to restore their souls. I'm not depressive, but in Lansdowne House and Port Hope, I was miserable. I checked, I guess, and the people weren't okay as I'd hoped. Had my father not been okay in the camps after all? Can a soul be nourished and sustained in a camp?

⊹ ⊹ ⊹

Telling people to take a trip was once a medical standby, a specific treatment for people whose souls need attention. "You need a rest [change of air, change of scenery]," said the doctors. I'm sure that, nowadays, although our methods may be different, doctors still tend our souls as ardently as they did a hundred years ago — and as ardently as a gardener tends his garden. Because in the modern world we think about our lifestyle, personality, and fulfillment consciously, we appear to have become a tribe of narcissists, overestimating what's personal; cultivating the personality and living life to the full are slogans on everyone's lips. Just the same, the soul, always at risk of being depleted or corrupted, needs restoration and refurbishing in every culture and every era. That's what I'm up to when I travel: my soul is restored if I see that people around the world are okay.

Psychiatrists like to institutionalize this notion, and speak theoretically of weak, alienated, estranged, or impoverished egos — not to mention fragmented selves, and the weak or absent superegos of psychopaths, all in need of soul-doctoring. One of the cures for souls is refreshment through seeing new sights, making new friends, and figuring out new ways of thinking. That's what happened to the souls of Odysseus, Dorothy in the land of Oz, and Alice when she went down the rabbit hole. But excursions entail risk; those who take drug trips may lose themselves in drugs or die, and Orpheus' trip to Hades to reclaim Euridice was a catastrophic failure.

We tell students they should go away to school, make a pilgrimage to Europe, undertake a modern version of the Grand Tour. Others urge unsettled friends to see a psychiatrist, leave home, go to military school, visit a spa, change their diet, join a club, find a faith, get out more, drink different water, take vitamins, go on a cruise. Often restoration of the soul requires mediation between different worlds: New Age space travel; yogic flying; commerce with the spirits of the dead; past lives; astrological influence.

These folk remedies have excellent credentials, and echo age-old stories like Persephone's annual trips to Hades, Little Red Riding Hood's adventure at her grandmother's house, Buddha's enlightenment under the Bodhi tree, Christ's forty days in the wilderness (not to speak of his death on the cross and rebirth on the third day), and Scrooge's journey to Christmases past, present, and future. And Cinderella, we know, went to the ball. Jail, too, for better or worse, inspires: Nelson Mandela and Adolf Hitler produced monographs while imprisoned; analogously, Cicero's writings on politics and philosophy flowered in exile. Other prisoners are damaged by confinement: Oscar Wilde, Egon Schiele.

To say the soul should be refreshed is, of course, an arousing metaphor, and like all metaphors, alludes to many quests. After ten years fighting in Troy, Odysseus took another ten years to get back to Ithaca, including a hazardous and terrifying trip to Hades to meet with the blind seer Teiresias, the only shade who (unlike the other shades, he'd been allowed to retain his capacity for thought) could advise Odysseus on how to get home. Odysseus' tasks and ordeals were the price he had to pay to find his way. Others undertake quests in order to reshape their identities, find their roots, or discover the woman of their dreams. Living in Egypt, for example, the biblical Joseph was cured of his self-destructive vanity.

Quests often include a crisis, the questors often urged on by healers who, innocent of what they're up to, induce death and rebirth scenarios: drug crises, insulin-coma treatments, and exhorting patients to "let go." *King Lear* is the story of a man who loses himself in order to find himself. I want to say the quest is universal, but generalizations about our species are risky. Like placebo cures, our mortal actions have family resemblances only to one another.

✢ ✢ ✢

In 1980, Nadira Persaud, who had just finished high school, was the summer replacement for my secretary. Nadira had been born in Toronto, but in the fall was going to the University of Rajasthan in

Jaipur. That fall and winter, I got letters from her asking for books; because books were in short supply, anything in English would do — paperbacks, junk novels. I rounded up unwanted books, plus books friends gave me. Nadira was starved for reading, and wrote further, asking for old *Time* magazines and, if possible, other magazines.

In a letter, I said to Nadira that one day I might show up in India. I got an enthusiastic reply: "Why don't you come this October, when my guru will be conducting an intense month of prayers at the ashram? People from all over the world will be coming."

I hadn't known Nadira had a guru; curiosity seized me and I arranged to go. First, though, I had to be vetted. Linda, Nadira's mother in Toronto, invited me to lunch to meet with her. Linda was worried that I might not be serious about my visit to the ashram, not a potential devotee. She asked anxiously about my beliefs and my morals, questions I neutralized with philosophical gobbledygook. I passed her tests, and was approved. "You must take this book and read it," said Linda. "It's written by the Maharaji." ("We call him Raji," Nadira had said one day with a giggle.) "You should also carry the book in your hand in the Delhi airport. Ananth, one of the Maharaji's assistants, will meet you, and if you have the book in your hand, he'll recognize you."

Later that night, I looked through the book; it was a list of clichés about eternal love and spiritual fulfillment. It also described the guru's years of sacrifice and lonely study, his quest, in other words, and his eventual recognition by the great philosophers of India as unique, gifted, and holy. His proper name was Jagadguru Shri Kripalu Maharaj.

Shamanic cults all demand spiritual trials and initiation rites. The psychoanalytic cult, too, is secretive, has initiation rites, and recognizes spiritual achievements. Like King Lear, prospective psychoanalysts must lose themselves to find themselves. All must be analyzed, a journey inward, so to speak, guided by those already anointed. Despite the absence of blatantly coercive brainwashing, there's no doubt we're a cult, although many friends will be annoyed by this statement and will dismiss me as a crank. Their claim will be that psychoanalysis is a science. They don't know that faith in the sanctity of science, be the believer a biologist or a psychoanalyst, is what makes us cultists.

Traditional psychoanalysts — and I'm one of them — think Jungians, Reichians, Rankians, Lacanians, and all other secret and semi-secret societies (Masons, Rosicrucians, Scientologists, Zoroastrians, Spiritualists, Occultists, Quietists, Futurists, Simple-Lifers, Utopian Socialists) are cultists, and so they are, each with initiation rites, adherents, and mysteries. Private languages abound: "The hypercathexis of the repressive drives . . ." instead of "He puts a lot of energy into kidding himself. . . ." Why is it bad to be, as I am, a cultist (a Freudian cultist, in my case)? Shouldn't cultists be judged on the grounds of what they actually do morally, as are stagehands and streetcar conductors? Surely spiritual worth is judged by a man's ordinary actions. Since we're all brim-full of allegiances, why not find interest and worth in what we are?

Cultists who live in uneasy association with one another populate every university department of English, philosophy, and psychology. We forget that the earliest philosophers — Pythagoreans, Platonists, Aristotelians, Stoics, and Epicureans — were not just adherents of philosophical systems, but members of organized schools, explicitly called sects. All such schools had "official" doctrines that, if not upheld, led to the expulsion of the dissident.

Our own cult is supposed to have the inside track on truth; we look on others as cultists, definitely not in the know. It's a sneaky trick we play on ourselves, unwittingly inching toward racism and prejudice. A good question would be why I, different from most people, am fascinated rather than appalled by my own cultish positions?

The answer is personal and, at least to some extent, has to do with having had minority status, being a German in Canada, during the Second World War. It wasn't like being a Jew or an Asian. Because my family didn't associate with other Germans, I had no group with whom I could play the malignant game I'm trying to zero in on, a game in which I could have joined a group and claimed, *We Germans are clean and industrious and sensible and thrifty, not like those Canadian ruffians.* It's the cure by hatred, and if I'd had the chance I might have joined in. Being on my own, I identified with Canadians just as much as with Germans, and became the arch-liberal. It's important to note the prefix "arch." Arch-liberals are fanatic liberals; they rant on behalf of liberalism.

✛ ✛ ✛

So, in 1992, I went to India. Armed with sneers and snobbery, I went to an ashram, which induced no crisis, and cured nothing, not even skepticism. I experienced only an amazingly different culture and utter boredom.

I landed in Delhi at 1:30 a.m. and, as had been arranged, Ananth — he seemed to be the guru's messenger — was there to meet me. So was Nadira. Ananth spoke English, although, as he told me, he was one of the few on the ashram who did. The guru spoke no English. We had a four-hour wait because we weren't starting the twelve-hour train trip to the ashram until 6:30 a.m., heading southeast from Delhi to a tiny village "near Kunda" in Uttar Pradesh, India's largest state.

On the last leg of our trip, a short hop by bus, I asked Ananth how to greet the Maharaji. "Just do what I do," he answered.

The ashram is in a village, the residents of which are part of the guru's flock, by birth assigned a destiny that excludes them from the formal religious activities. Their karma is to be labourers and farmers. The ashram itself is made up of a cluster of buildings, dormitories or apartments, and a meeting hall, where a party was going on.

The party celebrated the Maharaji. He sat on a platform — to me, it looked like a bed sprinkled with petals — and ate tidbits, some of which he tossed to the devotees crowded around. In two corners of the room were thrones, really heaps of elevated pillows, colourful, gilded with banners and gold edging. I noticed spotlights and strategically placed video cameras pointed towards the thrones. Every eye was on the guru. The devotees cheerfully bounced him up and down. Although it was a party, only the guru was partying; the others cheered and applauded as *he* partied.

He was brightly dressed, wore a large turban (only for the party), and shoes with curled-up pointy toes. Around his neck were garlands, and as he nibbled and shared his sweetmeats, the people threw flowers and petals. I was struck by his stature; he was the tallest man in the room, over 1.8 metres (6 feet), broad-shouldered and strongly muscled. Although he was over seventy, his thick shoulders were particularly noticeable, always shown off by sleeveless robes. Clean-shaven and handsome, his features were strong and bony.

I could see right away that the Maharaji's followers wished to make themselves — their souls — utterly subservient to him. Later, the devotees' thoroughgoing denial of their own interests — really a denial of their existence — became clearer. Always trying find in other cultures the rituals people use to cure themselves, I suddenly grasped that their self-cure was to have no soul at all, to shadow, ape, and adapt themselves to the contrasting soul of the guru, which was alive, vivacious, throbbing.

The party was ending as Ananth and I arrived, and shortly some of his followers helped the guru down from his platform bed. Ananth was clearly sorry he'd missed the fun, but he took me to the side of the room where the Maharaji was removing his turban and some of the garlands. Ananth threw himself to the floor and kissed the Maharaji's feet. "Just do what I do," he'd said to me on the bus.

I, too, threw myself at his feet, but did so carefully. There was no kissing. When I stood, the Maharaji made a joke, which was translated by Ananth: "It's good you are here. I'm the one who needs a psychiatrist."

I made a joke back: "Maybe we are in the same business."

He'd sized me up and instantly realized I was no devotee. The people surrounding us looked puzzled, probably because visitors were usually awed and submissive; my polite conversation probably looked irreverent. During my few days on the ashram, the Maharaji didn't pester me as he did the others. He nagged his devotees to take notes when he lectured, to carry their books, sometimes to come forward and dance. From the luxury of his thrones, he lectured twice a day, every word and gesture recorded by two cameras. When he and I passed, he acknowledged me politely.

Each day started at 4:00 a.m. with an insistent blast on a ram's horn; continuous chanting began and didn't stop until 11:00 p.m. Quickly, everyone gathered in the meeting hall for prayer and meditation, although the Maharaji didn't appear until later in the day. Most were poor Indians, although some were Indian immigrants who lived in Canada and the United States. There was an Australian woman, white, who'd had a bookstore in Sydney before moving to the ashram.

She'd been looking for a guru for many years, she said, and when she met the Maharaji, she knew this was the ashram for her. An American man, also white, was clearly a madman. He rarely spoke and stood in one position for many hours a day.

Several women spent the day cooking. Three times a day we lined up with our tin plates and were served the same bland food Linda had given me in Toronto: cauliflower, lentils, naan, yogurt. There was no meat or spices and nothing green. We ate with our hands, sitting on the dusty ground, a row of men on one side, women on the other. In the meeting hall, too, men and women sat separately.

Often, right after the guru's lecture, one of his assistants translated for three or four of us who spoke only English. At the translation session, the ideas still seemed silly, repetitive claims of peace and eternal wisdom for those who attended to the guru's message.

The assistant explained that the Maharaji keeps spiritual and physical things apart; he tries not to treat physical ailments himself. It is known on the ashram that he sometimes comes to devotees in their dreams and heals their ailments. It is unheard of to ask the guru for healing, because help comes by grace. Occasionally he cures people directly, usually by looking at the affliction fleetingly, by touching the body part, or by saying the name of the affliction or of the body part that is affected. Mostly, his cures are carried out secretly — secret even to the person healed.

The guru lives on behalf of his devotees. He parties, has a sex life, feasts, is married, and has children. They live vicariously. I watched the Maharaji go into a trance, peace and bliss in his face. And then, to my amazement, he had or mimed an orgasm: heavy breathing, glowing perspiration, pelvic thrusting. And bliss on his face. A few months later, in Toronto, I told my thoughts about the orgasm to Linda. "He was having an orgasm or pretending to have an orgasm. Do you devotees not see that?"

"Well, of course he was having an orgasm," she answered. "We live through him and he has to have orgasms on our behalf. Christianity is so impractical."

The Maharaji is the cure. The devotees have given up their souls and are reborn in him, like those reborn in Christ. But the devotees do it with a vengeance. In Canada, those who are serious about their faith know when the Maharaji has his daily bowel movement; they have theirs at the same time. He eats; they, thousands of kilometres and twelve time zones away, eat. He prays; they pray.

The devotees are examples of the cure by rebirth of the soul — but in this instance, reborn in their leader, not in themselves.

✤ ✤ ✤

Recreating one's soul, ardently and constantly, is universal. A bit of self-observation and any of us can see ourselves designing, revising, and perfecting the character we've decided we are. Every Friday, for example, I head for my cottage on Horseshoe Lake near Parry Sound. There I write, isolated from the city, imitating Philip Roth, Paul Gauguin, Saul Bellow, and all the others who've headed for open country to practise their craft. This placebo ceremony is one in which I twist myself — my soul — into another shape, a piece of vital nonsense. Many artists head for the city, of course. As reliably as at Horseshoe Lake, the south of France, or Tahiti, the soul can be re-engineered in cities: Paris, New York, London, Toronto.

When I head north in my car, there's more magic. Secreted in the back seat is a battered baseball hat, bought at Eddie Bauer. Its purchase accommodated the unique soul I've invented. It's from Eddie Bauer, you see, and not from a snobby shop like Saks Fifth Avenue or Holt Renfrew. Clearly, I'm a regular guy; this has been established and proven by where the hat was bought. It neither has a Blue Jays logo nor proclaims that I drink Molson's Export Ale. I'm plain, simple me, without fancy duds, but not joined up with popular culture either.

The hat transforms; as I head up Highway 400, I'm different, uninterested in showers and grooming, happiest wearing hat and baggy shorts. You can see that intense work is required to keep the old soul in tiptop condition. Establishing who one is must be negotiated with delicacy and finesse; a previous prime minister of Canada, Brian Mulroney, is still mocked because he wore Gucci shoes.

What about my unconscious? Well, it's not hard to figure out. I'm busy warding off the possibility that I'm a rich doctor, a snob who owns a cottage in the country, but I'm also not one of the masses. The hard work of keeping these two dangers at bay, looks like a fine case of humility and modesty, with a bit of fun thrown in, right? It's probably true, but it's something else, too. I want my soul to be that of an artist — badly. For a couple of reasons this shouldn't be public knowledge: first, it sounds too vain; second, I might fail, and what would people think? So I've conjured up a complex, repeatedly renovated soul for myself that covers all the bases. An extra gimmick that I've developed — a good one — is self-revelation, disarming and funny. Rediscovering the soul, you will have noticed, is a full-time job.

Weight loss, cosmetic surgery, assertiveness training, anger management — name any piece of your soul and someone will tell you how to reshape it. All placebo cures count on your hope, and mine, for transformation. Every *Bildungsroman* is about transformation: that's what *Bildung* means.

✛ ✛ ✛

Even rank amateurs have success with suggestion. Like many psychiatric students, when my friend John Robinson and I were residents, we experimented with hypnosis. We became good at hand levitation, but didn't get beyond that simple exercise. One morning before work, John came to my office. "I've got a toothache," he said. "I've been up all night and the dentist can't see me until noon, so I want you to hypnotize me and suggest the pain will go away until I get to the dentist."

Dutifully, I induced the version of a trance that John and I had practised. I suggested to him the pain would go away, that shortly I would refer to our supervisor, Bob Ortega, and, when I did that, he'd say he had to go. Before leaving, he'd check my window. Once out of the trance, he'd not remember what I'd instructed him to do.

"Are you seeing Bob Ortega today?" I said.

"Didn't work," said John. "You told me that I'd come out of it when you mentioned Bob and that I'd check your window. Also that I'd forget what happened. Well, maybe we'll get this hypnotism business eventually."

As he left my office, I asked, "John, how's your toothache?"

It had vanished. The only suggestion that worked was the one that mattered: that his tooth should stop aching. It looked as though my mystical suggestions had entered him, as it always looks with a placebo. Really, it was John's expectation, his wishful thinking.

The particular trick we use doesn't matter, as long as the healer is believed in, and as long as the procedure suggests potency: reorganize the energy field, practise exorcism, redirect the circulation by standing on one's head, kiss the tombs of martyrs and saints, wear amulets made of special substances, breath the smoke of burning herbs or burning goat's hair, use stinging poultices, ask for blessings, undergo electroshock, or tell your dreams. Stoicism, Epicureanism, skepticism and cynicism, psychotherapy, and antidepressant drugs work, too. "It works" is always the rallying cry.

I suspect that, when we circumcise our sons, tattoo our daughters, mutilate our genitals freakishly, and inject ourselves with dirty needles, vital ceremonies are being enacted. Jews are joyful when they circumcise their sons, as are Zulus when they tattoo their daughters. But when the ceremonies aren't time-tested, we are rightly skeptical. That's why it's best not to count on yogic flying, and safer to trust herbal remedies.

✛ ✛ ✛

In the corridor of the clinic where I work, I see colleagues chatting with their patients, often smiling warmly. Friendly chatter is the best way to silence patients: enthusiastic friendliness demands friendliness in return. How, I wonder, do they expect to get at the nasty bits of their patients, the sadism that intelligent scrutiny can unearth in any of us? When I watch such scenes I shake my head ruefully; although I'm a senior, I'm still Holden Caulfield.

This practice has been institutionalized in a psychiatric movement, "Integrative Psychotherapy," not time-tested, and unmindful of the complexity of human life. Instead of penetrating deeply, saying, "Tell me more," these doctors take their patients' statements at face value.

In my nightmares, these psychiatrists, dedicated to every known method of intervention, give patients whatever they ask for. Rather than seeking out their patients' most crippling truths, they quickly shower them with pills, advice, and referrals to various social agencies.

When patients up the ante, get more worried, pressure their doctors to "do something," too many doctors start worrying themselves, and resort to these weak practices. Many patients are glad to have doctors back away from deep scrutiny of their lives — patients are human, after all — and when psychiatrists dodge the nasty bits, patients are relieved. They're especially glad when, in the face of anger, psychiatrists placate them; no one likes to mess with his own malice.

Were the psychiatrists who placate their patients true integrationists, they'd also refer patients for bioenergetics, Christian rebirth, and colonic irrigation. Anyone can make such recommendations. A psychiatrist's job is different. If someone comes to see a psychiatrist, they've thought long and hard, the Aspirins and hugs of everyday life haven't worked, and it's time for more than banalities.

Always in character, I'm cocky and ready to fight when I hear that organizations open their arms to silly fads. I've pledged allegiance to a different caucus: a handful of colleagues; Wittgenstein and Nietzsche; my fellow malcontents. This is my folly, my very own foible, my way of surrendering my soul. But I'm doing my duty; what else can a doctor do if the caucus pumps out weak arguments about diseases? When the slogging gets heavy, I reassure myself with aphorisms. But I have to be careful, because aphorisms are too good to be true: there's an aphorism for every occasion, the best ambiguous.

✣ ✣ ✣

I'd seen the Maharaji make people happy, a sort of cure of the soul, but hadn't seen typical placebo cures on the ashram; apparently they were done in secret. The only place I'd had free access to shamanic cures was in the Mayan village in Mexico; in Africa I was pawned off on "tourist shamans," and the voodoo I watched in Haiti was suspect. In Ecuador I was assured there were plenty of shamans and that I'd be taken to see one, but nothing materialized. In Lansdowne House people claimed there were medicine men, but they didn't know who they were. "Someone told me he's the janitor in the school in Pickle Lake," one person assured me. But the Maharaji did have a major venture in the works — not a specific treatment but a mass healing of souls.

It was October 1992, and the Maharaji was about to embark on the greatest cure mission of his life, once again a cure of souls. This time it was offensive, a cure by hatred. The Maharaji and a group of his followers were on the way to Ayodhya, a dusty town on the Ganges plain, to visit Babri Masjid, a Muslim mosque. The mosque stood on a site considered holy by Hindus, although Muslims held it to be equally holy for them.

Little did I know the Maharaji was joining with three hundred thousand Hindus who, six weeks later, on December 6, 1992, would attack and destroy the mosque, originally built in 1528. That event sparked the slaughter of two thousand Muslims across the country. The justification? The mosque was (supposedly) on the site of Lord Ram's birth.

Whether the guru himself knew what was about to happen in Ayodhya is beside the point; the history of Muslim–Hindu violence is so much a part of Indian history that the Maharaji should have known better than to join with thousands of people visiting a disputed religious site.

I'm a loyal opponent of the cure by hatred, blaming the UN, the Muslims, or the United States — you name the enemy — but I'm less sure of my bravery. I ought to say I wish I'd gone to Ayodhya, where I could have been a moral witness. The truth is I'm relieved I passed up the chance. Even imagining what happened terrifies me, partly because of an experience I had after leaving the ashram.

Although the ashram culture didn't strike me as damaged like the culture in Lansdowne House, the Aboriginal community in Northern Ontario, it saddened me; worshipful devotion to the guru left out fun and adventure for the devotees. I'm cheered by two wisdom comments, the first made by Thomas Mann and the second by Miguel Cervantes:

. . . they and the whole audience espoused the view that rejection is a destiny like any other, with a dignity of its own. Every condition is a condition of honour . . .

We cannot all be friars, and many are the ways by which God leads his own to eternal life.

‡ ‡ ‡

I'd gone to a remote temple to see the uncovering of a black Krishna, which was exposed to fresh air and the public only every fifty years. There were thousands of us, and when I reached the entrance, the gatekeepers refused me entry. Only Hindus were allowed. Because I'm a pesky North American, I argued, and held up the line. There was a commotion. Because the crowd moved forward relentlessly, shoving and pushing, I was frightened, as were the gatekeepers. A fast decision was made to put sandalwood powder on my palm, which, in the same manner in which the host is taken into the mouth in a Christian church, I was then to put reverently in my mouth. A dot was placed on my forehead and, then a Hindu, I was allowed in.

When the black Krishna appeared, the crowd, packed tight, began to sway. No one could move, the swaying became extreme, panic set in. I thought I might die, but a dignified-looking man called to me urgently, "I'm Dr. Ganguli. You'd best come this way, Sahib."

In the side wall was a door I hadn't seen. The sign said "Europeans only." Dr. Ganguli and I went through and, like Alice, found ourselves in a special area — not a garden, but a quieter room uncontaminated by hysterical masses, where we were able to see the Krishna figure without obstruction. Meanwhile the masses swayed, sweated, and put their lives in danger.

I'm pretty sure that when I go to an ashram, to Burma, to Mayan villages, and other impoverished places, I'm checking up on my interned father, secreted in a camp resembling an ashram: dormitories, barracks, latrines. I keep concluding that they — and he — are all right, but I always have to check again.

PART THREE

PSYCHIATRIC CURES

CHAPTER THIRTEEN

EVERYTHING WORKS

PSYCHIATRISTS ARE DAMNED, CONDEMNED to adopt absurd mental attitudes, charter members of the cult of aliens and madmen — at best, respectable criminals. It's a hard fate and hard work; I'd been a psychiatrist for fifteen years before I did my duty and noticed something strange: most psychiatric patients get better regardless of diagnosis and regardless of what treatment they get. Drugs, humane support and encouragement, psychoanalysis, and psychotherapy all do the trick. This happy conclusion applies to every psychiatric category that's been devised — phobias, neuroses, psychoses, mood disorders. All psychiatric patients who've been assigned a medical label do well in the hands of psychiatrists of every stripe — *and in the hands of quacks as well.*

For years I'd faithfully attended Grand Rounds, the weekly educational meeting at my hospital, and heard the news about an increasing accumulation of discoveries, an arsenal of treatments that all worked, so many I eventually began to scratch my head in bewilderment. And all the studies shared the happy outcome: about 70 percent got better.

The most recent study I've come across,[1] on the treatment of depression, confirms that the results are still the same. Like many people, I'd been aware as a teenager of the mindlessness of passively accepting traditions, but over the years my awareness had faded, especially about the work I cherished, in-depth psychotherapy. Would my own method — analytic psychotherapy — eventually be flooded out by the barbarian incursions of temporary fads like phototherapy, cognitive-behavioural therapy (CBT), and the parlour-game methods of Gestalt?

One day in 1976, I heard of a new treatment for hyperactive children. Instead of treating the children directly, many families were brought together in a group family-therapy format, a kind and considerate business, I guess, that proved to work — just like everything else. I tumbled to the realization that I'd heard too many stories of treatments that "worked" and had the heretical idea that, if I treated people by requiring them to dance a jig in Piccadilly Circus or Times Square, that would work, too.

A research project added weight to my concerns. Difficult patients — most carried the spiteful title, "borderline" — were treated with a brief, twelve-session spell of psychotherapy. Many senior, highly experienced practitioners were enlisted to be the therapists. Most, including me, were psychoanalysts, skeptical that much could be accomplished in a brief treatment (analysts typically see people for dozens, if not hundreds, of hours). The patients did well, with a 70 percent improvement rate despite the usual expectation: they're not suitable; they'll have a bad outcome; twelve-session therapy is not long enough to help anyone. I began to think every treatment must have a good outcome.

What if, I thought, *all psychiatric treatments are just a placebo effect?*

Except, of course, this couldn't apply to *my* way of practising psychiatry. My way is traditional psychoanalysis, not slipping into modern revisions. Modern innovations in psychoanalysis, I noted, are infected by superficial fashion and all want to retreat from the deeply searching tactics of psychoanalysis.

❖ ❖ ❖

The test was whether I could turn doubt on myself, and speculate about the placebo nature of the changes wrought by my own work. Could it be true that my hard work only made people feel better because they believed in me and my ways? Could it be that my inspiring teacher, Karl Menninger, when he taught us psychoanalysis, believed in a cure that was bogus? Bogus is a harsh word; if both parties to the analysis act in good faith, shouldn't their efforts earn a bit of honour? On the other hand, and disconcertingly, Hitler certainly, and Saddam perhaps, acted in good faith. Siren voices beckon to us all: parents, religions, teachers, revolutionaries, art, and conformists all tempt us with their songs. God help us if, when the tempters beckon, we don't instruct our sailors to tie us to the mast. If not, we'll fling ourselves into the arms of a lovely sea-nymph whose song wafts in the winds — and who'll petrify our bones. For many years Freud was enthralled by the siren with the shining hair — her name was "Cure" — but late in his career drew back from disaster; he wrote a skeptical paper called "Analysis Terminable and Interminable."

Despite my claim that the good effects of psychiatric treatment are due to the placebo effect, the word placebo is seldom heard in the halls of psychiatry — except when referring to the sugar pills that, in research studies, are compared with real drugs. Psychiatrists are a sanguine lot, rarely think about the placebo effect of their own treatments, and are remarkably magnanimous about one another's treatments. Psychotherapists obligingly agree that drugs are helpful; biological psychiatrists reciprocate by acknowledging the good effects of psychotherapy.

But I know a secret: drug people are convinced the only valid treatment is psychopharmacology and covertly scorn psychotherapy; psychotherapists, in private, just as sure that only their psychotherapeutic practices yield worthwhile results, scorn those who rely on drugs. The exception is the eclectics, the psychiatrists who believe in everything — except they go pale when I ask them if they believe in faith healing, Chinese herbs, acupuncture, aromatherapy, bioharmonics, crystal power, homeopathy, and reflexology. A true eclectic would, obviously, go along with such methods. Although eclecticism is fair and liberal, the world is too multi-faceted. We're stuck with having to choose.

Non-psychiatric doctors are more interested in the placebo effect of their treatments than are psychiatrists, a generosity they can afford because their usual job is to treat biological abnormalities. They have treatments with objective, curative effects. When evidence accumulates, they can see they've sometimes been wrong and freely acknowledge that certain of their cures were produced by the placebo effect. Unlike psychiatry, other branches of medicine have objective tests — blood abnormalities, X-rays, physical signs — that clinch whether or not abnormalities exist or have been corrected. Psychiatry has no objective tests. This is not a relative statement: the number of objective tests a psychiatrist can rely on is zero. To contradict the last statement, someone would have to give an example of an objective test for psychiatric disease.

✢ ✢ ✢

At dinner the other night, my friend Doug Frayn told our table about Buddha's teaching that, "pain is inevitable, but suffering is optional." George Boujoff, another friend, smiled. "Mark Twain," he said, "had something to say on that subject: 'I have suffered many terrible things, some of which may actually have happened.'" These are fabulous pieces of wisdom but, because they imply that people can choose to do otherwise, the aphorisms don't apply straightforwardly to the modern world's hypochondriasis; it's hard to change one's thinking about precious things. What is clear is that scornful commentators like me ought to pull in their horns. Through illness, these unhappy people speak, commenting on their lives in code. Humans have always done this, but in the modern world, the language has changed.

Once people spoke of sin; they confessed, beat their breasts, and wore hair shirts. The perception of personal wickedness was rampant, as rampant as the perception of illness today. The change is in our articles of faith: once we believed in God and the Church; now we believe in Doctors and Science. In the seventeenth century, suicide was called a sin. Not only were suicidal sinners condemned to damnation, but their corpses were attacked. Stakes were driven through their hearts, their bodies were dragged face-down through the streets, they were buried in insulting locations.

By the nineteenth century, most suicides were declared *non compos mentis;* the language had changed from sin to illness. Both attitudes illustrate human intolerance; few people are willing to say suicide (and madness of all kinds) is merely one of the amazing, enigmatic things people do. Those who reflexively assign puzzling behaviour to the mental-disease category think they've become humane, but I suspect this terminology is a euphemism, an excuse for our determination to exclude from the human mainstream those whose unconventionality makes us uneasy. If we say they have a mental disease, we're saying they are damaged members of the species.

Life is a struggle, excrement rains down, but that's not what we say; we speak in our culture's favoured language. For example, in Lansdowne House, the Aboriginal community I described in chapters 7 and 12, people insisted that an accidental death was caused by a snowmobile and not by the careless driver. A hole was sawed in the ice and the snowmobile was dumped in. These particular Aboriginal people, it seems, are good Platonists. In the *Laws*, Plato proposes that, because it carries a miasma or pollution, an animal or inanimate object that causes the death of a man should be tried, condemned, and banished beyond the frontiers of the State.

The cultural dogma current in Toronto says otherwise. The accidental death is assigned to a different category; the drunken driver of the snowmobile did the killing, so he needs either to be treated for his alcoholism or charged with a criminal offence. At least that's how we're *supposed* to react. I no longer get to vote on such matters because, baffled, skeptical, and a cultural relativist, I no longer know what causes anything.

When I told the Ojibwa of Lansdowne House that, in Toronto, when there is a car accident, the driver of the car is held responsible, they were amused.

✥ ✥ ✥

I'm making a radical claim: modern hypochondriacal complaints are religious cries, shouts of guilt, the modern equivalent of hair shirts, self-flagellation, and making our hands bleed with the stigmata on Good Friday. These cries appeal to a new religion — Science — that aims to cure but has another task: to reconnect people to their culture. Or, better: by way of medical and scientific rituals, through thick and thin, Healers and Doctors celebrate with patients their membership in the culture. Doctors and Healers have always been granted "priestly" status, and as a result have carried both respect and power. The measure of respect has grown; doctors are the new priests. They offer benediction, and speak in a mysterious, ceremonial language, offering plenty of talk about therapy, with big words, Latin words. "You've got *erythema multiforma*" only means the patient has funny-shaped red blotches on the skin. On the rare occasions when I write prescriptions, I still write them in Latin (with some Greek symbols thrown in), thereby evoking a splendid placebo effect. Both alternative and traditional medicine are, in the best sense, performance art.

Not everyone is satisfied with traditional ceremonial practices. Yoga and Tai Chi, for example, practices that spring from distant cultures, are the enthusiastic choice of many Westerners. Those who practise these arts are getting straight who they are just as singlemindedly as those who feel better participating in traditional Western medical ceremonies; some like to settle their identity by way of Eastern disciplines. They are announcing, both to themselves and others, that they aren't standard issue.

Clergymen know their counselling role has been diminished, passed on to psychiatrists and other therapists. Every psychiatric hospital I've worked in has had student clergymen pursuing training in psychotherapy. They know well, but not clearly, that the modern word is "treatment."

Recently a psychotherapist left a message on my voice mail. "Don't be surprised when the receptionist says this is a funeral home," the message said. "I'm also a therapist and a grief counsellor." Shades of *Six Feet Under*!

What most offends those who don't agree with me is when I say the placebo effect is first cousin to a magical or religious ceremony. The word "ceremony" shocks and offends them, which means it won't easily come into popular use. The term doctors insist on is "treatment." Is it possible we could be dead honest and call it a placebo effect? Probably not, because that word names the magical element too nakedly; those who wish to believe their treatments are real, will believe, evidence be damned. Try explaining to a believing Catholic that praying doesn't seem to do anything, and you'll see what I mean. The word placebo smells too fishy.

Although these matters are part of ordinary human life, I worry. I can't do better than to quote the brave words of Ivan Illich, cultural critic, philosopher, priest:

> [The] medicalization of health beyond a certain intensity increases suffering by reducing the capacity to suffer and destroying the "community setting in which suffering can become a dignified performance."

The placebo effect can be put to good ends; therefore it's part of excellent medical practice. But it can also do mischief. Whether it's good or bad has a complicated answer, and depends on the method and spirit in which a procedure is delivered. Once we had a paranoid and obsessive belief in the right to salvation, and churches saw to it that we got it — or so we thought. Nowadays, we have a paranoid and obsessive belief in the right to health, and doctors see to it that we get it — or so we think. Oftener than not, our right to health is delivered as a placebo. We also think we have a right to wealth, freedom from misfortune — when the goddess Fortuna fails to smile on us, we file lawsuits — and a right to insult suffering people by calling them mentally diseased. Mostly, those who suffer those insults at our hands are just unconventional.

CHAPTER FOURTEEN

CHANGING THE THEORIES WE LIVE BY

I'VE INSISTED THE PLACEBO EFFECT IS DUE to suggestion, but that neglects the interesting puzzle of how or if people change deeply, the exciting thing that makes for good movies and novels — and if it doesn't happen, the stuff of tragedy. King Lear and Cordelia change, but not soon enough. I'll admit, as I've insisted throughout this book, that we're safest if we stick to saying, "Change is just one of the things people do." But an important topic can't be dismissed so quickly. I'll start with a digression, an examination of the nature of science, the often-abused method through which we devise practical theories of the world, often with fabulous payoffs. Although we are not scientists, we psychiatrists also have practical goals: to discover how to help people change.

The scientific method isn't rarified or unusual. In truth, it's something we all do: it's the method of "trial and error." Watch a youngster use a computer or hook up a stereo system. More boldly scientific than an adult, he guesses that this button, this arrow, or that box ought to be clicked, and, with the stereo, plugs in wires here, then there — experimentally.

With lightning speed, he's building hypotheses, subjecting them to the test of functionality, and rejecting hypotheses that don't work. That's what scientists do. In contrast, a technician follows a manual.

When it was hypothesized that the Earth rotates around the sun, the theory was tested. Experiments that were designed to falsify the theory were tried out, and when all the tests were done, it was accepted that, yes, the Earth does rotate around the sun. Theories that survive experimental tests take their place in the academy of scientific theories. They are true, *for now*.

If, later, a test disconfirms an accepted theory, the theory falls under doubt. This goads scientists into testing the theory afresh, aiming to settle once and for all whether it can be kept in the stable of confirmed theories or must be discarded. If it fails the tests, new theories have to be dreamed up to replace the one discarded. That's what the boy at his computer is doing — building hypotheses, testing them through little experiments, discarding those that fail, and finally sticking to the one that works.

An infant, watched closely, can be seen early on to conduct similar experiments. Because we live according cultural roles, habits, rules, and rituals, it's a skill an infant can't do without. It's what defines us as human.

"Here I come! Here I come!" I said one day to my granddaughter. I lifted her up, kissed her, and wrapped her in a bear hug. She squealed happily. On my knee, she reached for my glasses. I stopped her and, with mock anger, scolded, "You rascal . . . don't you dare take my glasses . . . I'm going to bite your tummy . . . monkey . . . funny imp."

She kept grabbing. Several times more I told her to stop, each time more sternly. Finally, only slightly chastened, she stopped.

A bit later, at dinner, she reached for a camera lying on the table. I said firmly, "No!" She looked closely at me, and, still looking at me, tentatively reached again for the camera. I said again, "Mariah, noooo . . ." She gave up.

When she reached for a forbidden object a second time, Mariah was conducting an experiment. She already had a hypothesis in mind: "I'm not supposed to touch the camera. 'No,' means I have to stop." Like a good scientist, she subjected her hypothesis to a test. My second "No" confirmed that her theory was right.

When, without evidence, hypotheses are clung to, we're no longer in the realm of science. Instead, we speak of faith, the obvious example being religion. Religious speculation has nothing to do with science, and anyone who tries to subject faith to experimental tests has missed the point: Gods and rituals are grounding philosophical positions, axioms to live by, so to speak. Axioms, even in science, don't get tested.

Because it is a certificate of decent citizenship, proper and respectable, belief in God comforts many people. In intellectual circles, other points of view are what give comfort, faith positions as axiomatic and dogmatic as religion, such as materialism or capitalism. Because it certifies that he is a respectable intellectual, being a skeptic, a relativist, a nihilist, and an anti-foundationalist, comforts many scholars in a postmodern world.

More to the point is to consider the hypothesis that psychiatric disorders — madness, depression, suicide — are biologically caused. In science, if a theory is not confirmed, scientists lose interest; it gets forgotten. The ancient Greeks hypothesized twenty-five hundred years ago that severe madness had biological roots. Yet, strangely, and despite millennia of non-confirmation, the theory persists, as we saw in Chapter 2.

Why would that be? The answer is this: the belief that psychiatric disorders are biologically caused is a faith position, an ardently believed-in ideology, first cousin to any other axiomatic or religious belief. This makes the hypothesis neither good nor bad, but only settles that psychiatry's scientific claims are rhetorical props, unsubstantiated by evidence.

Despite its shrill voices, the anti-psychiatry movement does its small bit to change things. I'm nervous that my unorthodox views will lead my colleagues to think that I'm in cahoots with these anti-psychiatry organizations — "weirdoes," "paranoids," "crazies," as they get called by established psychiatrists like me. They won't, we say, leave decent psychiatrists in peace as we do our good work.

My fears expose my vanity, my readiness to posture as one of the good guys, a member of the establishment. I ought to be soothed by anti-psychiatry's achievements, accomplishments, real political effects: recently, the movement's pressure on the American Psychiatric Association resulted in a press release in which the association admitted that no abnormal biology for psychiatric disorders has ever been demonstrated. Tucked among many paragraphs of careful filler, the American Psychiatric Association conceded that:

> Still, brain science has not advanced to the point where scientists or clinicians can point to readily discernible pathologic lesions or genetic abnormalities that in and of themselves serve as reliable or predictive biomarkers of a given mental disorder or mental disorders as a group.[1]

This should not be a surprise. But I wish the American Psychiatric Association had reacted like the scientists they claim to be, eagerly interested in critique and clarification. Why in the world would they equivocate by saying, "has not advanced to the point," "readily discernible," and, "in and of themselves"?

Once, the strange, the odd, and the bad were sinners, another faith position that, in a world as crazy then as it is now, gave solace and comfort. Searching out solace and comfort is natural, but science has nothing to do with feeling better. If we're baffled by the folly, unhappiness, and craziness of our patients, we're wrestling with something that resembles the meaning-of-life dilemma. Psychiatrists must be clear that, yes, they do and should build theories and have hypotheses. But they also must keep in mind that their hypotheses, valuable or not, have nothing to do with science. Psychiatric theories, very important, serve a different purpose: they soothe the soul.

Faith theories, be they religious or psychiatric, work only if they avoid getting literal, detailed, and rational. There's no harm in saying, "God help me," and there's no harm saying of my crazy aunt, "It's a sickness with her." But once we take faith positions literally, make them rational, we slip into prejudice: those who don't believe in a specific God are then our inferiors — infidels, pagans, and sinners. The same goes for psychiatry: literal claims of disease define patients as being our inferiors, those with defective brains, abnormal chemicals, destructive genes. The psychiatric faithful have become equally prejudiced. If, some day, it's proved scientifically that God exists and that depression is biologically caused, I'll have to eat crow — but I'm not worried.

It's wonderful that, in the zodiac, we see a ram, a lion, and a crab, and just as wonderful that, in the same zodiac, the Chinese see a rat, an ox, and a monkey. In our hearts and souls, all are real. I'm a Leo, but if I believe that I'm really and truly a lion, I'm either stupid or bonkers. The fallacy of literal belief is a far better definition of a delusion than the traditional one, which holds that, if a belief is culturally wide-spread, it's not a delusion. The nasty conclusion would be that, since in 1939 it was widespread to think Jews were an inferior race, prejudice against them was okay.

The belief in lesser people is, I'm convinced, the most important of the psychiatric disorders. The lesser-people delusion is not officially a disease, largely because, rather than being in our patients, it's in us, the practitioners. Like other unofficial diseases — epidemic greed and international paranoia, for example — its study is neglected.

When one raises doubt about beliefs, one often hears cries of "You're nothing but a nihilist." People who say this haven't paid atten-tion. A proper nihilist doesn't deny meaning; indeed, he insists on a *plurality* of meanings. A beautiful woman may be a collection of mole-cules, but it's far more important that she's a goddess, the girl of my dreams, and the stuff of poetry. Stephen Vizinczey, novelist and liter-ary critic, author of *In Praise of Older Women*, once spoke of "the kind of barbaric incomprehension that would describe a woman's glance by saying she has twenty-twenty vision."[2] Any materialist who insists that the *real* reality of the moon is that it's a lump of rock has set aside the visions and dreams that matter.

✛ ✛ ✛

Understanding why life is edgy and painful depends on understand-ing important things about the mind, how each of us builds up his view of the world, what we call psychology. Destined from birth to live in a culture, people develop hypotheses about how to fit in, then test out their theories. Here is an invented example of how this might happen:

Cordelia, like Snow White and the Sleeping Beauty, believes —'it's her hypothesis — that she is the best-loved child. When her father, King Lear, divides up his kingdom and, without qualms, intends to give her the lion's share, her hypothesis is confirmed. Cordelia decides that to have become the best-loved child — she is Lear's baby — has been unwise, improper, and harmful. Aiming to devise a new strategy on life, she goes back to the drawing board. Perhaps, she thinks, a better strategy would be crankiness, to not go along with false declarations of improbable love. She tries it out, declines to say her father does, and always will, rank highest in her love.

This new hypothesis about how to live a life serves Cordelia well – for the moment. It solves a problem for her: her guilt over being the best-favoured. The strategy of ill-temper doesn't work either, of course, although it is disconfirmed only over time. Late in the play, Cordelia finally understands that crankiness, impertinent honesty — she'd made a nasty scene at an important royal ceremony — is also cruel honesty, that perhaps her ideas about how to live still aren't as good as they could be. She revises things again, this time in a change of character that is one of the most dramatic in English literature. Literal honesty, she realizes, is trumped by humanity. When Lear tells Cordelia that he now knows he has wronged her, that she has "some cause" to hate him, she demurs. Having added graciousness of spirit to her repertoire of life strategies, she speaks a noble lie: "No cause, no cause."

Cordelia has changed. Like a scientist, she is willing to revise her theories and has become a different person, better, wiser.

✧ ✧ ✧

The human species has developed the ingenious trick of not having to conduct experiments in nature. We do it in our heads. It's the human specialty. Other animals think, try things out, solve problems, but unlike humans, it's not their specialty. Elephants, dogs, and monkeys certainly learn and figure things out, but their thinking isn't as central, so defining of what their species is. The experiments we conduct internally, in our minds, are modelled on what goes on in nature, on the hard lessons and trials of evolution. In *The Blind Watchmaker*,[3] Richard Dawkins uses the example of cheetahs and gazelles.

If the genes of a newborn cheetah program it for extra speed, it will grow into an adult better equipped than other cheetahs to catch gazelles, feed on them, and survive. Chance (The Blind Watchmaker) periodically produces such cheetahs, who, because they are particularly adept hunters, survive better and produce more offspring. Slowly, over the millennia, the inheritance of the new, speedier characteristics will predominate. Over time, cheetahs get faster.

Gazelles evolve in complement. Those who run fast, have better colour disguises, and develop escape tricks, get hunted down less frequently by cheetahs, hence come to predominate. It's the law of the jungle, survival of the fittest.

I'm making an analogy. Cheetahs and gazelles, by passing on diverse assortments of genes to their offspring, are doing experiments. Each cheetah and gazelle born is, so to speak, an experiment, conducting a test to see whether this genetic variant or that will survive better. It's the living world's experimental method. When a variation leads to greater success, new traits — speed, disguise, evasive tricks — come to predominate. The genetic experiment has been subjected to tests, not in a test tube, not in someone's mind, but in the field.

Since most genetic variants work badly, experiments in the field — "Is this a better way to hunt (trick, hide, escape)?" — tend to fail. Variants that fail, if they don't disappear instantly, fade from the gene pool quickly. Only successful experiments survive. The analogy to psychiatry is that, having failed all tests (no physiological abnormalities have ever been demonstrated) biological theories of psychiatric disease ought to disappear — fast.

That psychiatry's biology hypothesis hasn't faded shows that it is ideological, not scientific. But it is badly managed. A worthwhile ideology would recognize "biology" as an important and evocative metaphor; instead it's treated as literal truth. Biology is a valuable metaphor, because it increases our linguistic versatility. Once we've got it in mind, we can say things like "Her hormones made her do it," or "That jerk needs a new brain." But I'm not stuck with biology. I can also say "He's nothing but a kid" (a double metaphor, child and baby goat), and "She's full of beans," and "He's another Jack the Ripper." But any metaphor believed in literally is a delusion, including the delusion that trouble, self-torment, and weirdness are diseases.

Since gazelles are designed to elude cheetahs, and since they get better and better at this every generation, there is evolutionary pressure on cheetahs to evolve, too — in the direction of better hunting. And since cheetahs are equally brilliant in design and self-improvement, there's equal pressure on gazelles. No evolutionary change takes place unless there is pressure on the species to change.

Analogously, Cordelia won't change unless there's pressure. The same goes for a psychiatric patient. Since his madness or suffering is based on his self-devised theories about how best to function in his culture, community, and family, without pressure to rethink his assumptions, he won't change. I assume that living in a culture, a community, and a family includes being under plenty of pressure. This is exactly what's called for.

It's risky when genetic changes are extreme. If cheetahs evolve too far in the direction of speed, they may use up resources at the expense of something else. Dawkins's example is milk production. If leg length, muscles, and speed are developed at the expense of milk production, extra-fast cheetahs will die out. Interestingly, in the psychological realm, there is no such limitation. That's why changes in thinking and behaviour can be fast, profound, unexpected, and peculiar. Psychological experiments, even radical ones, aren't usually lethal.

Some ways of life — experiments — lead to lower reproductive rates, for example homosexuality and "schizophrenia" (extreme madness is the term I prefer). People with these ways of life have fewer children, so their genes are underrepresented in the gene pool. Yet, despite low reproduction, homosexuality and madness don't disappear. This is because such ways of life are psychological styles and have nothing to do with genes. Any person may end up designing himself to live in one of these ways. No genes need apply.

The human element that is genetic is our imaginative minds. Those bequeathed a genetic program that produces strong muscles, a pretty face, and good digestion receive no benefits from their attractiveness if they can't negotiate the culture skilfully. To live in a culture requires us to figure things out, build hypotheses, and come up with theories that have been tested by experimenting with life. But life must challenge us.

It's been known for years that babies in orphanages who are washed, fed, and kept warm don't thrive.[4] Many die, and those who survive are often developmentally delayed or handicapped. Parents and families are different from an institution; they stimulate infants, make demands, offer things. The necessary ingredient is parents who are a presence, lively, and recognizable as unique. In an orphanage, the caregiver is anonymous; a child assigned the same caregiver every day does better, but not as well as one who lives in the hurly-burly of a home.

Parents don't just care for children. They are unpredictable, have moods, yell and kiss, laugh and joke. The caregiver who tends the baby in an orphanage does these things, too, but in that setting, her interesting qualities are muted, dulled by institutional life. In institutions there's no stereo blaring rock 'n' roll, nor is there a dog who poops on the carpet, a cat yelled at for leaping into the crib, or a crowd of cooing relatives.

An infant has no choice but to contend with the buzzing kaleidoscope he lives in. Around these images, the building blocks out of which he constructs a world, he weaves hypotheses: this is who I am; that's who I'll become; I think that's what that person is like; this is what the world is like; this is the best way to negotiate this messy place. Identification, we psychiatrists call it, an ingenious, self-designed amalgam of the cultural images by which the child has been impressed. Challenge awakens us, makes us think. And when we think, we build hypotheses and test them. However, apart from arguing about them, I don't know how to put these ideas to the test.

The final word on scientific work aims to psychologize it, make clearer that the mind is concerned with thinking, not with tangible experiments in the material world. The hypotheses I've described are actually internal narratives. For example, it is common to say that

Columbus discovered America, a Eurocentric narrative hotly disputed by anyone who has thought about it. Arnold Toynbee tried out something a bit different: that history is a record of challenges — climate, nutrition, war-like neighbours — to which nations and tribes respond in one way or another. Traditionally, historical writings have been guided by stories of leaders, royalty, and wars, the master narrative we always thought was plain truth. Modern historians try out other narrative guides: the history of disease, for example, or of art, baptismal records, or army-admittance forms. New narratives make history look different.

Each of us has a set of master narratives. Two common psychiatric "master narratives" are: all behaviour can be reduced to biology; you get in trouble if you don't ask patients about suicidal tendencies. Less-common psychiatric master narratives are: traumatic events and improper parenting cause people to be sick; discrimination against women (people of colour, immigrants) is not adequately taken into account by my male (white, Anglo) colleagues. The master narrative of psychoanalysis is that ardent listening reveals the truth. This hasn't lasted, and has been replaced by reductionistic narratives like: all psychopathology is caused by the Oedipus complex; madness is due to defects in the ego; symptoms are due to libidinal fixations.

Left out are the real psychiatric narratives: literature is the best template we've got for human behaviour; all actions are culturally embedded; psychiatrists nudge people towards a more comfortable cultural niche; the personal narrative of the patient steers us in the right direction; the hidden purpose behind personal narratives is the key to understanding.

⁂

The need for pressure was driven home for me when, in 1971, I left the native community of Lansdowne House and, on vacation, went directly to Haiti. François Duvalier, "Papa Doc," was in ascendancy.

I'd been appalled in Lansdowne House to discover the people had lost rudimentary skills like bathing. The factor at the Hudson's Bay store cashed the mothers' welfare cheques. On sale in the tiny, one-room store were furs, but it was hard to tell who would have bought them. The mothers gave bits of money to their children, who, also at the Bay, bought food: chips, Cokes, cans of beans, Spam. Their mothers didn't prepare food.

The men hunted, but wouldn't go to the hunting ground unless a government plane gave them a lift. They were losing their skills: travelling, tracking, transporting game.

In Haiti, all was different; social assistance didn't exist. On the way into Port au Prince, the bus stopped because a water main had broken. The women passengers got out of the bus, took off their children's clothes, and bathed them. Once done, they hoisted up their skirts, washed their legs and feet, then their faces, necks, and arms.

On the streets, I was under attack; vendors, hustlers, money-changers pestered me. The culture was impoverished, vibrant, and noisy. To survive, people had to be busy and industrious. They were also happy. At bus stops, early in the morning, people, singly and in groups, hummed quietly and danced.

Although idealistic to a fault, I'm not fool enough to wish Haiti's culture on Lansdowne House. I'm out to make only one point: challenge, pressure, danger, and instability are necessary for change, and the Ojibwa of Lansdowne House were under no pressure to adapt to their changed world. I'll remind you of this when I suggest ways psychiatry might do better.

✦ ✦ ✦

Shouldn't the pain and suffering of psychiatric patients be a stimulus, a prompt, a motive for change? Surprisingly, the answer is no. There are two reasons why not. First, if they are convinced that they have a disease, it induces passivity; what can one do if it's a disease? The second reason why their own disquiet doesn't prod psychiatric patients towards change has been discussed in Chapter 3, that symptoms, though painful, symbolize a solution better than any other they can imagine. The important thing to keep in mind about this point is that psychiatric symptoms are a compromise. They are the best the patient has been able to come up with, a compromise that keeps at bay ideas and feelings that, to the patient, seem worse than their symptoms. This is misguided, perhaps, but, since we all have fears, obviously true.

And we're not talking only about avoiding obvious things like shame, humiliation, and anxiety, because many of our fears are unexpected. Sometimes, for example, the fears are about things usually thought desirable: achievement, fame, and sexual fulfillment. Whatever the fear, our patients solve their dilemma by adopting a small evil, one they deem safer than the imagined greater one. For example: "It's better to think and live as a harmless, depressed drudge than to think that, like Snow White and Cinderella, I humiliated my mother."

Like all of us, Cordelia practised the suffering-to-avoid-suffering manoeuvre. By arranging rejection by her father and expulsion from her homeland, Cordelia eluded something she feared more: triumphing over her sisters. To her, triumph was more to be feared than rejection.

✤ ✤ ✤

When patients are treated, they feel helped. If, for example, a depressed man is given a tonic, he'll soon report that he's better. Additionally, something has prodded him, challenged him, shaken his usual way of thinking: he has been certified as sick, told he requires treatment. Before, he wasn't sure, but a new status implies rethinking who he is. "I'm a depressive kind of guy" is replaced by "I have a disease."

I don't like the "You are sick and need treatment" message, but, just the same, it will prompt a patient to shed previous ideas — hypotheses — about who he is. Had this depressed man been given electroshock treatments, it would be more dramatic. "Wow," he'd think, "whatever it is I've got calls for really strong measures."

If given Prozac, he would be warned about side effects, further drama, fuel for the placebo effect, just as regular blood tests would impress on him that something important was happening. The patient's thinking is what's affected; his previous way of understanding himself is challenged. The more dramatic the intervention, the greater will be the challenge to his established world view.

Chaos theory agrees that complex systems can suddenly change, often after tiny alterations in conditions (I'll hold my nose and agree to use the language of "people are complex systems"). Stock markets, storm systems, and chemicals, stable until a small, critical change takes place, suddenly fluctuate wildly: the stock market crashes, storms break out, and a chemical reaction takes place. Insofar as it reacts to symbols — the death of the president, for example — the stock market resembles humans who, responding to symbolic cues, divorce, commit crimes, or change careers. This phenomenon has also been called "the butterfly effect."

But I'm not convinced the interventions of doctors are more arousing than the events of everyday life. Life's tests and challenges are more unsettling than any tonic, pill, or shock treatment could be. The complexities of love, sex, loneliness, and career, more than anything else, inspire us and drive us mad.

There is, of course, a treatment that purports to promote major personal change: long-term talking therapy, also called psychoanalysis, dynamic psychotherapy, or in-depth psychotherapy. Psychoanalysts are convinced that only unremitting, long-term pressure can lead to substantial change. Other psychotherapies, cognitive, behavioural, interpersonal, don't have this aim. They are designed to get the patient through a rough patch or to put aside symptoms. Since long-term psychotherapy is my specialty, I'd like to convince you that psychiatrists like me help patients to make real changes in their style of life.

CHAPTER FIFTEEN

PLACEBO: THE SECRET HEALER

THE BOY TOLD THE DOCTOR THAT SOMETIMES his knee hurt, but at other times was fine. At school, about to run a footrace, his knee would ache, but he could make it better by shaking his leg. The boy (clearly a budding psychiatrist) wondered if it might be bad nerves — sissy nerves. The doctor examined the knee and found nothing wrong. "It's growing pains," he said.

It was 1943, and the eleven-year-old boy was me. Dr. Broad was our family doctor and, earlier, had made a house call to see my mother. My knee was a side issue, but those simple words, "It's growing pains," kept me from worrying about my knee for thirty years. I jogged, played sports, and climbed mountains. My growing pains always responded well to a bit of shaking out of the leg.

In 1973 the knee wouldn't work any more. I limped and couldn't drive my car for more than forty minutes without stopping and walking around. And shaking it a bit. My surgeon, Peter Welsh, flexed and extended the knee, twisted it, and put his ear close to listen to its creaks and clicks. "The medial meniscus is damaged," he said. When I awoke from surgery he said nothing had been left of the cartilage but a tangled lump, that grooves had been worn into the articular surface of my tibia, and that I must have injured it thirty years ago or more. "Don't you remember?" he asked.

My mother had the answer, and echoed the surgeon's words. "Don't you remember?" she said. "Three big boys carried you home from the hockey rink because you'd hurt your knee."

I remembered. During most of those years, orthopedic surgeons had only reluctantly opened knee joints to repair them, but it didn't matter because, for thirty years, my knee worked, a cure based on the placebo magic of three words: "It's growing pains." Dr. Broad had given me a sensational gift.

Dr. Broad was a family hero whose only truly medical-technological service to us had been managing the difficult birth of my older brother who, at three months, died. He didn't charge us during the Second World War, because my father had been interned, and he knew there was no money.

I eavesdropped carefully during another of his visits when a different side issue was discussed — not me that time, but my Aunt Dona, who'd become paranoid, something I'd noticed on my own but, at age eleven, had concluded was just her typical nuttiness. Clearly, I was already a Wittgensteinian: *That's just what she does*, I'd thought. I guess she'd got worse and announced to us that, on streetcars, people whispered about her. At first this was ignored, but later the family worried, because Dona became preoccupied and could talk of nothing else.

Dr. Broad had a brief answer to the family's inquiry about what might be going on: "She's having a nervous breakdown. Didn't you have a nervous breakdown a couple of years ago, Anna [my mother]? She'll get over it just like you. She really ought to stop working for a few weeks. Isn't there another sister in Halifax who she's close to? Why doesn't she go to Halifax for a couple of weeks?"

And so she did. When Dona got back, her suspiciousness was still around, but she was calmer, and after a few months the whole thing was forgotten. I have a hunch that, nowadays, Dona would be given antipsychotic medication, but have no idea if this would have speeded up her recovery.

After we finished our psychiatric training, my friend John Cody moved to Hays, Kansas, to run the local mental-health centre. He taught his staff — and his patients — that the people who came to the centre were having nervous breakdowns. He'd just graduated from the Menninger Clinic, world famous and academic, but he used none of the high-falutin language that defines people as suffering from diseases; he told them they'd had nervous breakdowns.

. ✤ ✤ ✤

I have a third example of simple, magical cures, this time of *group* anxiety. Once again, the cure was linguistic, worked by the use of a single word, a cure I couldn't have performed myself, because it happened in Germany at a time when I couldn't speak German. It was a dinner party during *Fasching* (*Karnival, Mardi Gras*) in Frankfurt am Mein and everyone — costumed, dancing, singing and drinking — was having a wonderful time. We were in a public hall and I was disconcerted when someone at a nearby table fell to the ground. I was a doctor, so I had to do something but without language my doctorly powers were crippled. Had I needed to, I wouldn't have been able to say, "Growing pains," nor could I have said, "She's having a nervous breakdown," or, "He's fainted." In medicine, common things are common, so the odds were that it was a faint, but if I'd had a look and decided that's what it was, I wouldn't have been able to say so.

As I walked towards the man lying nearby on the ground, I was relieved to see someone else step forward, his confident manner making it clear he was a doctor. Quickly he examined the stricken man. The crowd surrounding him anxiously waited for his verdict. Finally he stood up. "*Kollaps!*" he announced. All heaved a sigh of relief. How peculiar and yet how obvious. The word had the power to explain, to reassure, and to bring the disturbing event to closure.

I worry these stories won't hit home, that many doctors, especially psychiatrists, won't see the profound bearing they have on how we practise. They'll understand Dr. Broad and the German doctor weren't doing technical or scientific medicine, and that their manner and speech delivered indispensable symbolic messages, but they won't see that *all* psychiatric practice is one or another version of delivering symbolic messages.

✢ ✢ ✢

Patients have to play the doctor–patient game with us; they'll benefit from ceremonial treatments only if the illusion they are invited to join in on is one that has interest for them. If they don't, it messes things up just as much as when doctors don't do their job. Patients who don't believe in doctors, don't come. The illusion of the useless or terrifying doctor suits them better than the more traditional illusion, respect for doctors. Medically, such illusions are costly, because, as well as selling dreams and illusions, non-psychiatric doctors provide biologically curative treatments.

Many patients visit doctors, then mistrust the doctor's manner or what he offers. One man felt enraged at every doctor who gave him advice. He saw only pomposity, arrogance, and arbitrariness. But he visited doctors and usually — not always — followed their advice. What bothered him was the vulgar self-assurance of doctors, their grotesque confidence in raw facts, clear solutions, and their expectation that their instructions would be obeyed. This man, a patient of mine with an artistic bent, admired performers and people of refined culture.

His mother, also of an artistic bent, had similar fits of fury at doctors, but did *not* follow her doctor's advice. When told she was having a heart attack, she was outraged, flounced out of the emergency department, and the next morning was found dead in her car in the hospital parking lot. My patient knew his mother had, in effect, killed herself, but couldn't shake the idea that his mother had been right to be annoyed at the doctors. For him, there *must* be an external devil.

One patient of mine attended a meeting of breast-cancer victims and pumped her arm in satisfaction when she reported what had happened. As she listened, another woman told the group what she did when her surgeon had told her she had cancer of the breast. "I slapped his face," she'd said. The group cheered and applauded. It's one of the strange, self-invented placebo cures, the comfort of finding someone to blame, even when knowing the blaming is misplaced.

※ ※ ※

It's one of the distinguishing features of psychiatrists that we stick by angry patients without placating them or explaining away what happens. But, in the real world, and despite what I've said, psychiatrists internally react like everyone else. As often as not we're impatient and judgemental, except we're good at keeping our poise and thinking about what's going on. One of our less attractive tricks is when, occasionally, we kick out difficult patients by finding an excuse. The patients belong, we say, to a dead-end category. They are "borderline," or have a "character problem."

I believe that, if psychiatrists feel unable to work with a patient, they ought to be plain-spoken, not make excuses or candy-coat their message. They ought to admit that the problem is theirs, that they can't work properly any more. If they don't, they are just silent farters.

> Oh, the shark has pretty teeth, dear
> And he shows them pearly white.
> Just a jack knife has Macheath, dear
> And he keeps it out of sight.

Sharks are honourable, says Bertolt Brecht; they show their teeth. Silent farters are worrisome, because their weapons can't be seen.

I'm suspicious of words like "borderline" and "character problem," but have my own self-deceiving method of being a sneak, squeezing out difficult patients in my own way. Despite liberalism, altruism, and endlessly bleating that I'm determined to help, I'm as much of a coward as anyone. I'm sure that my tone of voice, body language, and the messages oozing out of my pores, one way or another, tell difficult patients to get lost. I'm never explicit, but a few will get the message, a message that, even as I send it out, is safely secret. Blinded by fake virtue, I don't have to feel guilty, nor can patients complain. Just the same, part of me says: "You're not wanted; get lost; you're hopeless." Shakespeare taught us we're *all* liable to be sneaks and excuse-makers.

My placebo organization demands that I hang on to a particular philosophical conviction: that every reality — mine or anyone else's — is an illusory set-up for understanding the world. Don't misunderstand. By illusory I don't mean false or silly. I'm saying that every way of understanding the world is an illusion, a psychological "construction." Some are common, so conventional and widely shared we don't see them as illusions. Others are uncommon, therefore judged bad, silly, or mad.

My own illusion includes the idea I'm talking about at this instant, that I've got to keep in mind that reality is always a personal construction or illusion. If I succeed, I can cling to my idea that the world isn't just craziness. My reality and every reality can then be seen as tentative, as art and performance. I have smart friends who think this is baloney, that I'm nuts. Well, I am.

But they are, too.

✦✦✦

Like the advocates of tough love, most of us think that, in the long run, reality breaks through. I listened once as a group of patients decided that it was good to stay in a difficult marriage ("it's reality") because difficulties lead to personal growth — a reminder of my musings about how change is only possible in the face of challenge or provocation.

Even great epics err on this point, often arguing that material reality must win out. Odysseus, dining with the Phaeacians, made witty conversation about the belly's power. He'd fought in Troy for ten years and for ten years more struggled to get back to his home in Ithaca. No matter how beaten down, he said, hunger and its greedy organ, the belly, insist and demand to have food. The reality of hunger trumps all misfortune.

As he tells the story of Odysseus, Homer shows us that he agrees. Instead of using chapter headings, Homer punctuates with repetitive, ritual statements. *The Iliad* and *The Odyssey* are divided into sections by tangibles: food and time. It's a decree: reality punctuates the world. "When they had put aside the need for food and drink . . ." and, "When Dawn once again spread her rosy fingers across the sky . . ." The realest of realities are, it seems, eating, the gods, and time.

Marlowe, Joseph Conrad's narrator in *Heart of Darkness* makes a similar claim. In the face of hunger, he says, "superstition, beliefs, and what you may call principles, they are less than chaff in a breeze."

Biology agrees. In essence, the human body is a tube, one end a mouth, the other an exit. All other organs are auxiliary: sex organs for creating new hungry tubes; oxygen collectors, lungs, used to burn food; liver and pancreas to help out the gut in its digestive work.

But Odysseus, Homer, Marlowe, Conrad, and biology are wrong. Amazingly, even though from a biologist's point of view we're glorified tubes, a person will die for a cause, a rag, or a principle — starve to death for honour or appearance. In fact, it is principles, our illusions of what counts as ultimate value, that trump all.

Here are life goals, pedestrian, preposterous, and ordinary, as varied, mundane, and strange as yours and mine. Odd goals are as valid as the conventional ones we all know about: marriage, career, money, going to movies, having hobbies, raising children. We judge oddness, fail to remind ourselves that peculiarity only matters if it hurts someone. Those who are odd get called crazy — legitimately perhaps, but it doesn't mean they need a doctor or a hospital. It's hard not to laugh, love, or be repelled by:

- The autosex expert, who aims to be the finest masturbator in the world.
- The passionate lover of poetry.
- My acquaintance who does cryptic crosswords and belongs to the corresponding international organizations.
- Someone who joins MENSA.
- The well-practised man who has become skilled at producing fine stools, encouraging his bowels to be thorough, enthusiastic, and whose products are richly coloured and aromatic.
- Donnie Eisen, gourmet cook.

+ Bill Clinton (or Arnold Schwarzenegger), devoted to being loved by everyone.
+ The professional fool: Mike Myers, Jerry Seinfeld.
+ The park-dweller.

To tolerate all visions of the world is liberalism, a non-judgemental attitude towards even bizarre ways of life, an impossible tolerance. Such liberals, against every instinct, realign their minds and decide that things usually called nuts, crazy, and a mental disorder are just odd and unconventional. Such liberals, psychiatrist or not, stand against people hurting one another, but for them these are moral and legal problems, not psychiatric ones. They also worry about those intent on hurting themselves, but fear their nervousness might lead them to interfere with a person's rights. Best, they assume, to consider individual cases.

✤ ✤ ✤

Lawyers often ask psychiatrists to see their clients, but often they shouldn't agree. If clinicians, they can only say that what the person does or thinks is a product of the illusions by which he or she structures his or her life, which is what psychiatrists can say about anyone. They *could* say certain behaviours are conventional or non-conventional, common or uncommon, but that's not what lawyers want; that judgement can be offered by anyone. What's wanted is the certification of normality of abnormality, judgements psychiatrists can't make — unless they've switched from being psychiatrist to self-deceiving moralist. As Thomas Szasz has said, "Medicine uses pathologists to prove disease; psychiatry uses lawyers!"

When we do this, mistake moral judgements for pathology, we've decided such a patient has inferior health, not to speak of an inferior disease. Declared to have diminished responsibility, he's no longer a moral agent. Transgressions are then not to be penalized because, being incompetent, the patient is not responsible, not fully human in other words. Disguised as consideration for someone ill, his or her social dignity has been stripped away. The *secret* healers have disappeared: an arbiter of humanity has taken over. Healers are "secret" because their help is magical, embedded in interesting rituals, always benign. They amputate no limbs, organs, or pathology, nor do they amputate civil rights.

There's an old empirical dictum: *natura non fecit saltus* ("nature does nothing by leaps and bounds"). My illustration of this is that madness is no further away than the reflection in your bathroom mirror, your family in the kitchen, your next-door neighbour, or the characters in any television drama.

Despite the experts, it's just not possible to decide that Jack knows the nature and quality of his actions, and Jill does not. The only honest judgement is that Jack's actions are odd or wicked and Jill's are not. In addition, and in accord with common sense, Jack's or Jill's personal statements about what they understand don't count either; any child caught with his hand in the cookie jar might say, "I wasn't going to take one." Self-deluding as we are, not even our private beliefs are conclusive. Were Jill not a moral being, she could be only a pre-programmed robot or a blithering idiot.

The alternative to calling immoral behaviour "pathology" is not blunt retaliation. But measures taken in response to actions, punitive or not, must keep in mind that patients, children, and criminals are entitled to the dignity of full citizenship.

If a madman says he screams at night because the Freemasons, the Socialists, or the Terrorists torture him, a psychiatric pathologizer will listen, but disagree about the identity of the terrorists. He agrees there are torturers, but doesn't believe the miscreants are moral offenders. With as little evidence as the madman (none, in other words) he will tell the court that the offender, madman or not, is mistreated by Free Chemicals, Socially Maladaptive Genes, and Terrorist Synapses. These imaginary internal offenders are the grounds for deciding the patient is no longer a moral being.

⁜ ⁜ ⁜

In modern courtrooms, as often as not "abnormal" could be expressed by the statement, "My syndrome made me do it." Be it murder or shoplifting, the accused claims he or she has a disease: battered-wife syndrome; alcoholism; nymphomania due to Prozac; borderline (antisocial, inadequate, narcissistic, impulse-ridden) personality; post-traumatic stress disorder; multiple personality. In the modern world, I ought to say psychiatrists who testify to such things are ill and suffer from court-testifying syndrome.

I'd like to find an excuse for my colleagues, but because I suspect many believe the silly things they say, I can't. If psychiatrists become legislators of morality, they've abandoned their medical contract with our culture: treat disease and disquiet, make no judgement. Saying a human action is pathological is a slick but dishonest way of saying something is bad. Cancer and asthma are pathological, but not morally bad; hallucinations and phobias, however, are *not* pathology, but share cancer's status as not morally bad. If, when hallucinating, a man kills, it's not pathology, but it's certainly bad. "Don't judge mental habits," says the real doctor, "only judge deeds."

Any psychiatrist who doesn't understand this point should immediately cease practice and sign up for the infantry.

We need social policemen, but the law and courts have been assigned that job, guided by constraints and obligations that protect people who come under their jurisdiction. My position — radical in the current psychiatric culture — is that mental pathology should only be diagnosed if it's clear the doctor is using a metaphor: "This woman is sick (a mess, a nervous wreck, a nut case, a worry wart), and may want to talk to a psychiatrist." Doctors who decide they have discovered actual diseases distance themselves from what they see. They cure themselves — not their patients — by putting them in a "class." Emily Dickinson could definitely be talking about psychiatrists in this poem:[1]

> I pull a flower from the woods —
> A monster with a glass
> Computes the stamens in a breath —
> And has her in a "class"!

To say a person is a psychiatric case is quite another matter. This is never a moral judgement, only a decision that the person is suffering psychologically and might (note: "might") want to see a psychiatrist.

Because it invites us to be helped, the illness model has advantages. But the model is threatened by bad theories and bad thinking. It's certain that a medical problem isn't synonymous with biological abnormality. Were biological causes of psychiatric troubles ever discovered, they'd be treated by family doctors and internists, and psychiatrists would disappear.

Although ill, psychiatry isn't suffering from pathology. It would be politic to say the illness is ordinary and human. It's closer to the truth to say psychiatry's illness is error, bad navigation, carelessness.

CHAPTER SIXTEEN

RADIANT ODDNESS

IT'S EASY TO TEACH PSYCHOTHERAPY: TELL students to give advice, pronounce moral judgements, and follow a manual. Because we can count on the placebo effect to make patients feel better, these juvenile approaches to human suffering will work just fine. The psychiatric debate is not, and never has been, about how to make people feel better; that part is easy. The debate is about medical influence, which goes far beyond help given to individuals. Doctors are powerful models for how worry, unhappiness, and madness are to be understood, and for how suffering might be relieved.

Advice, judgements, and manuals all suggest there is a right way of living a life; they are moral edicts. I say: leave moral guidance to families, friends, and self-help books; they boost us up when untidy life gets us down. But this has nothing to do with finding the right way. Ostensibly, moral counsel aims to get people to behave better — once in a while we all need to be told to behave ourselves — but when friends counsel us, as often as not, we've coached them into giving the advice we want to hear. The job of friends is to soothe us, by gabbing, gossiping, sharing a bit of indignation or a joke.

Besides, there's a moral injunction for every taste. If I advise calming down, the psychiatrist in the next office might well advise the expression of feelings. Other examples are easy to find: standing up for one's rights versus compromise; marital fidelity versus following the longings of the heart; calling a spade a spade versus valuing one's job.

It's a sure bet that psychiatrists — they should know better — have advised both sides of every pair I've named. Life, I'm afraid, is too complicated for such recommendations to be anything but harmless chitchat, wholesome and necessary when we lean on friends and family. But for those not helped by home-spun support, psychiatrists owe a higher wisdom. A *lot* higher.

The ceremonial practice called psychotherapy is an offshoot of a well-known medical skill, the good bedside manner, a skill indefinable and unteachable, practised badly by some, expertly by others, and improved only by a teacher's inspiration and plenty of clinical experience. Be it good or bad, all doctors have a bedside manner, a ritualized style as important as the specific treatments they advise. For psychiatrists, rituals are a specialty. Like all rituals, psychotherapy thrives on mystery and the unexpected.

✣ ✣ ✣

A few days ago, just before 11:00 a.m., I sat in my office waiting for Jane Clement, the patient seen with a group of students and described in Chapter 7. Among other things, she'd had a gagging problem. After that meeting, I'd decided I would work with her in psychotherapy myself.

Mrs. Clement comes twice a week and was due any minute. When my watch signalled 11:00, I walked to the waiting room and nodded silently. Ahead of her, I walked to my door, stopped, and waited as she walked in, crossed the room, and lay on the couch. I walked to my chair, which is behind the head of the couch, and sat down.

After a minute or so, Mrs. Clement sighed and began to talk. "Nothing's new. James [her husband] is so stupid. I told him again it was time for us to split up, and all I wanted was money for the bus fare to Vancouver, where my girlfriend lives. As usual, he said he had no money, but the next day, when the truck broke, he had money to get it fixed. He says he's going to Sudbury next weekend to play in some hockey tournament. He has plenty of money. He just doesn't want me to leave. I don't want the furniture or the truck or anything, just enough money to get to my girlfriend's place."

She fell silent. I've heard these complaints before, and know she doesn't intend to leave. She often has money, which leads to a recurrent theme: she doesn't want to initiate any actions. Leaving her parents' home is the only act of initiative I've heard about, and even that was a simple switch from her parents' safe nest to her husband's. She knows she avoids initiative, but ignores the theme, especially since she knows it's linked to her father's sexual abuse. Like many abused women, she fears that signs of initiative mean she'd been an initiator with her father.

"I guess I'm a homebody," she said, "so I can't leave. It's weird. After leaving my horrible family, you'd think I'd find it easy to leave now."

The word "homebody" didn't seem right, but when she said it, a song suddenly ran through my mind.

"A song has flashed into my mind, Mrs. Clement," I said. "It's an old navy song. I'm not sure how it fits with what you're saying, but let me sing it to you."

> She had a dark and a roving eye,
> And her hair hung down in ring-e-lets.
> She was a nice girl, a decent girl,
> But one of the rakish kind.

This is not common practice. I've sung like this three or four times in my thousands of appointments with patients, and its rarity, and my usual sober style, make the ritualized nature of my work all the more obvious. When I do things like this, I don't talk about it, afraid people will think I'm barmy.

Mrs. Clement giggled, then checked her giggle and launched into a sneer: "You're always so polite, but you're a prick like all men. What a stupid song. You've probably got some smart-aleck interpretation for me. I come here to get help, but I don't get much. Why would you waste my time horsing around like that?"

I stayed silent, another important psychiatric ritual. Besides, anything I said would have been a trick aimed at soothing her: explanation of the meaning of the song; explanation of why I'm silent; encouragement to think about the song and what she imagined I might have in mind. Rituals, designed to encourage thinking, are the stuff of the cure.

Her outburst was followed by silence, which I eventually broke by dryly adding the following: "When we were teenagers, we didn't say, *And her hair hung down in ring-e-lets.* What we sang was, *And her hair hung down between her tits.*"

"You really are a boor," she said. "That's exactly what I expect of guys. You're such a phony."

More silence.

"You're determined to be 'a nice girl, a decent girl,' and never to be the rakish kind. It's your safety trick. You won't wander away from your husband because if you did, it would mean you're a woman of action. And you decided years ago that you'd never be a woman of action. If you did, you'd think you were a woman of action at another time in your life, a terrible time. You've spent your life designing an image in which you never act, and the stuff from the past, you'll never talk about, although you're content if *I* talk about it. In other words, I take verbal action and you don't; someone else took action when you were a kid, and you didn't. That's the message you're trying to get across, but it's a cover-up. It's a cover-up of what you secretly fear, that way back then, you were the person of action, that something about you or what you did, made those things happen.

"Do you know why I don't say it straight out about the bad thing that happened years ago, name names, and describe and name deeds that were done? It's because I don't want to play the game where you don't talk about things and I do, where you're passive and I'm active, where I'm rakish and you're just *the nice girl, the decent girl.*"

"Well, it's just that it's too horrible."

"[Softly] *She was a nice girl . . .*"

"Cut it out. Give me a chance."

"*And her hair hung down in . . .* Yes, I mustn't pressure you to commit the deed of action. I'm to shut up and leave you with your illusions. [Even more softly] . . . *a decent girl.*"

She stayed silent again, musing about her fear that any action would be incriminating.

"Definitely not rakish," I said. "Not an explorer and adventurer like Little Red Riding Hood. If you were, you'd think you were the one who seduced the wolf."

"Oh, shut up."

"Huh? If I shut up, your game would be ruined. I'd be inactive and the ball would be in your court. We've got it pretty clear by now that your favourite trick is to always be the inactive one."

"You don't have to get sarcastic."

"Well, now that you mention it, I *was* getting sarcastic, which means we've switched roles. Yes, I see what's going on. It's what you noticed, me taking over the sarcasm. Usually it's *you* who's sarcastic with guys. The best example was when the dog bit your husband's nose and lip and when you drove him to the hospital you made wisecracks about what a jerk he was. When the intern first interviewed you, she commented on it. Did she use the word sadism? I can't remember.

"If we're switching roles — me getting sarcastic instead of you — the next thing you'll be talking about you-know-who doing you-know-what to what's-her-name when she was a child."

"I know," she said. "I guess we've talked about this before, too. But I'm sort of stuck. I don't know what to do."

I was tempted to point out that, once again, she was "stuck," but figured that would be nagging. Hammering home a point doesn't promote thinking — only submission or opposition. Besides, I'd already been far more talkative than usual. After two or three minutes of silence, the appointment time having run out, I said, "Our time is up."

She stood up silently and walked out, caught up in the automatic rituals of ending. Had I reassured or encouraged her, she would have let me know she understood the rituals of ending; she would have called me a prick again, and she would have been right.

✤ ✤ ✤

What has happened? Does Mrs. Clement have a disease? Certainly she is miserable, uncertain, stuck. I could say she's unhappy and, since she gets crabby easily, it's sort of a "sickness" with her, but that would be a metaphor. I could just as well say she's a bitch or a wreck — more metaphors. Like all metaphors, the words would point to things that are poetically, rather than literally, true. I'm no more scientific if I say she's a suffering human, but I'm pointing at something important.

You may have noticed she doesn't sound disturbed. Surely, you might say, she's just talking about the ups and downs of everyday life? I risk putting the necessity of my profession in jeopardy if I say that, if we listen, all our patients talk about the ups and downs of everyday life. Like grand opera, psychiatry is about what's common to all of us. But there is more to people like Mrs. Clement than meets the eye.

Another question would be whether I'm curing my patient, thus drawing an analogy with diseases that can be cured. Mrs. Clement would almost certainly say she's better, but she'd also say she feels better when she has her hair done, visits her friend in Vancouver, or drinks a martini. Visiting a friend and going to the hairdresser make us feel better because, like psychotherapy, they are placebos; unlike psychotherapy, drinking a martini, as well as being a ritualized ceremony, is a physiological sedative.

✤ ✤ ✤

Psychotherapists offer a "cure" that's intrusive; we stick our noses into our patient's habits. Courteous, professional, measured — but persistent. When patients say they are sick, we're polite, but in our hearts know we will butt in, pressure them to notice their harsh judgements of themselves. These are most apparent when they use euphemisms, purport to suffer from some form of pathology when they really mean to insult themselves, to tell us they are improper, unworthy. All psychotherapy patients wrestle with guilt, none more than those who think that psychological disquiet is sickness. Psychotherapists won't have it.

To illustrate that moralists, their patients' blood brothers, are to be found everywhere, psychiatrists might well remind self-judging patients of moralists like George W. Bush and Billy Graham. Such moralists worry psychotherapists, a worry they need not hide because they are fine illustrations of how, by blaming others, humanity can go off track. Psychotherapists often use as examples the most terrifying moralists of all: Adolf Hitler, Josef Stalin, Mao Zedong, and Pol Pot, fanatics driven by evils to which they themselves were blind.

The struggle against judgement doesn't end with a final answer, a cure, because every "better way of looking at things" turns out to be another judgement: "Ah, I judge that now I'm thinking about this better." Psychotherapists tease apart good/bad attitudes as they come into play in the consulting room to demonstrate that moral positions are worth thinking about, that good and bad aren't as obvious as they seem. Hurting or humiliating people pretty well sums up what counts as evil. Greed, peculiar clothes, believing in astrology, gluttony, or weird sex, and being a social isolate, although often judged, don't matter much.

Insofar as they deny final truth, psychotherapists are nihilists, insisting instead on many truths, all needing consideration. Because nihilism demands that we doubt our own habits, psychotherapists acknowledge that thinking about different truths, those that go against our instincts, is hard and painful.

✢ ✢ ✢

Children don't learn about lovemaking by watching in the parents' bedroom, and students of psychotherapy don't learn by watching in the consulting room. The deep importance of these vital human acts thrive in solitude and mystery. Both are learned in bits and pieces, through nudges and winks, and by watching how those we love interact with the world. The final flourishing of lovemaking and psychotherapeutic skill depends on the practitioner's native wit; he has to figure out the details himself. Lovemaking is a work of art, and the sex act its subsidiary attribute. Practising psychotherapy, too, is artistic, "technique" mere detail.

The public purpose of my seminar at the university is to teach dynamic psychiatry; my private purpose is to inspire students to think like me. This is embarrassingly vain, but it's the truth. The alternative would be to teach students to think like the psychiatric profession at large, a way of thought that — to put it mildly — worries me. If I'm lucky, a few students will become thinkers; I hope all will rethink the standard patter. Students won't pass their exam if they think like me, but I'm incorrigible; I don't want them to be unthinking apes.

✧ ✧ ✧

In Goethe's and Thomas Mann's versions of the Faust story, when he was tempted, Faust knew the devil's secrets before he heard them, uneasily aware his conservative good sense was in jeopardy. And in both versions, because familiar with the ideas, Faust suspected the devil was a figment of his own imagination. Like all provocateurs, I suspect that I, too, am a figment of your imagination.

Although some will disagree, I'm firm on this point; we all think widely, flirt with devilish blandishments. It's hard to imagine someone not smart or curious enough to worry about the issues I've brought up. I'm skeptical about people not being smart; the psychologically thick are portraying themselves as "not getting it" just as ingeniously as those who, convincingly, sell themselves as clever, mad, benevolent, or criminal. Every trait and every madness is a role, so well rehearsed we forget that, for the benefit of both the world and ourselves, they are portrayals of who we are.

"Portrayal" conjures up stage acting. But an actor plays his part temporarily, although, if portraying Cleopatra, an actor may, tongue in cheek, "become" Cleopatra off stage. And innocently, in ordinary life, that actor may become Cleopatra unwittingly, an act which will amuse, surprise, or annoy those who know her. But, like the madman's portraying himself as mad, and unlike the actor, the person who "isn't bright" doesn't play out his social role temporarily. Unless he's got an abnormal brain, being a dimwit is his career, deemed a deep truth, just as it's deemed a deep truth that I'm critical and that Jesse James was a crook.

Not being smart or curious is not an existential state. As far as I can tell it's another habit of living, the most amiable compromise a particular person has been able to devise. It's strange perhaps, but so are the habits of bums, gamblers, and drunkards. Supposedly "stupid" people are geniuses at making sure no one could imagine them to be clever.

A vested interest in their jobs couldn't stop psychiatrists from having doubts about the practices of their profession, but they might nevertheless avert their eyes. Some researchers do avert their eyes; others know clearly that they tweak the system. Lots of skilled investigators, working under the banner of psychiatry, make neuro-physiological discoveries that have wide medical importance — even when their findings have nothing to do with psychiatry.

Simple conservatism has the same blinding effect as "not getting it." The redactors of the Judeo-Christian Bible, in the service of protecting the faith, suppressed the Bible's original exciting and subversive ideas. It is the unquestionable duty of traditionalists to smooth subversive thinking; conservatism is common and normal. But it should *not* be common and normal in academics and scientists. When conservatism afflicts psychiatrists, they've stopped paying attention, both to the nature of science and to their patients. If they did pay attention, it would be obvious that society is an association of minorities, not a melting pot into which all must fit. The weird, odd, and crazy may or may not want to fit in. To a heterosexual, a gay man's sexual preference may seem odd, but he can't be asked to "fit in," to become straight; it's a contradiction in terms.

✤ ✤ ✤

Although often under suspicion, doctors are determined healers. I've scrubbed in with surgeons, amazed at their scrupulous thoroughness. Breast cancer, for example, tends to spread to nearby lymph nodes in the armpit and, even when the cancer had surely spread widely, I remember surgeons diligently dissecting out tiny nodes, just in case they might be able to remove every last cancer cell. *Curb your enthusiasm*, I thought. A terminal case of fatalism, I inwardly shook my head in amazement — and admiration. That's why I couldn't have become a surgeon; its exacting demands would have been beyond me. Yet, in my psychiatric work, I'm as stubbornly persistent and indefatigable.

My colleague Gerry Shugar recently referred a young man who, after assessing him, I began seeing in psychotherapy. The patient was depressed, and for many months had been unremittingly determined to kill himself, urged on by violent fantasies of how he might do this. Outside of the safety of a hospital, working with such a patient is frightening, yet, without a second thought, I went ahead. The hazard is less that the patient may kill himself — we all know this can happen — but lawsuits and the harsh disciplinary eye of professional colleges loom in the background. When there's a complaint, it's a gut-wrenching nightmare, causing weeks and months of sleeplessness. Consequently, since professional colleges don't stand behind their membership as they once did, doctors outside of hospitals are skittish about seeing such patients.

The other day I passed Gerry on the street. "Hi, Gordon," he said. "You took on that young man. Only you and I are crazy enough to take on such cases."

"We're doctors, for Christ's sake," I answered.

Gerry's eyes narrowed and he smiled grimly. There was a silence, both of us thinking the same thing. "Somebody's got to treat a kid like that," he said.

"Gerry, that's why I hate it when people throw around that 'borderline' bullshit all the time. I think it's an excuse to not to work with tough cases."

"Exactly," said Gerry, then added, "Thank God you and I are perfect."

Gerry is not perfect, nor am I, but we've accomplished something that matters; neither of us has theosophical convictions about psycho-analysis or biology. Whatever our delusions, we're not enthralled by the common things that could distract us from being doctors. Why do we do it? Because we're caught up in the traditional doctor role: attending to pus and blood, piss and shit, suicide, hatred, violence, and craziness. Having bought into doctoring, we have no choice but to do that job. It's not virtue, just a crazy passion that possesses us. Like lovers, psychopaths, and evangelists, we're consumed by a social role. To be a bum, a lout, or to join the cult of victimhood is, just as ardently, to occupy a social role.

A lot of doctors are like that. Some of my colleagues in psychiatry, when a patient doesn't get better easily, try drug after drug. Their folly makes me shake my head in disappointment; yet I never stop trying my own methods. And when doctors have tried and tried yet again, they finally bring out their best and heaviest weaponry: placebos.

His diagnosis, stated with all reserve, was of something like a stomach ulcer, and while he prepared the patient for a possible hemorrhage, which did not occur, he prescribed a solution of nitrate of silver to be taken internally. When this did not answer he went over to strong doses of quinine, twice daily, and that did in fact give temporary relief. But at intervals of two weeks, and then for two whole days, the attacks, very like a violent seasickness, came back; and Kürbis's diagnosis began to waver or rather he settled on a different one: he decided that my friend's sufferings were definitely to be ascribed to a chronic catarrh of the stomach with considerable dilatation of the right side, together with circulatory stoppages which decreased the flow of blood to the brain. He now prescribed Karlsbad effervescent salts and a diet of the smallest possible volume, so that the fare consisted of almost nothing but tender meat. This treatment was directed towards the desperately violent acidity from which the patient suffered, and which Kürbis was inclined to ascribe at least in part to nervous causes — that is, to a central influence, the brain, which here for the first time began to play . . . spared light . . . ice-caps . . . consultation with a higher authority . . .[1]

The patient, Adrian Leverkühn — Thomas Mann's Faust — disagreed with Dr. Kürbis and thought that, if only he could meet a mermaid, a sea-maiden who, out of love, would trade in her lithe and muscular fish tail for a pair of painful legs — in other words, if his pact with the devil were fulfilled — perhaps then he'd be helped. Like all of us, Adrian didn't want to know he was under the devil's influence, in thrall to the cloven-hoofed, red-assed tempter. But science hates such talk.

✢ ✢ ✢

I'm still in Domaine de L'Étoile. This morning, July 12, 2003, I'm sitting outside having breakfast. The big day has arrived, and this afternoon in Vence my son Karl is being married. After working on this book for many months, I now see placebo cures everywhere, happy rituals and ceremonies that wed people to the world just as my son will be wed to Jill later today. I'll weep in the church, because that's what I do, but a more satisfying answer, one that makes me feel wise or cleverly analytic, is that for me, a tough character, a tear or two will add texture to who I am, disarm those who think I'm stiff, and, without becoming my difficult mother, I'll be a sentimentalist. Analyzing stuff, you see, is another one of the things I do. By now, you'll know that "what someone does" is a code word for "how people heal their souls" and for "placebo magic," the trait that so fundamentally defines us as humans.

I know from what happened at last night's pre-wedding dinner that, after the church service, five-year-old Tom, the Vietnamese adopted son of two of the guests, will joyously court twenty-five-year-old Angel, the best man's girlfriend. We'll all be charmed by Tom's innocent passion, but he'll pursue Angel too long and too ardently. The other guests, Angel —she's young and gentle — and Tom's parents will get uneasy. Little Tom is, you see, in love with Angel; he can't be distracted, can't stop touching her. And Alexander, Tom's father, will

eventually do his job, lay down the law, face Tom with the harsh realities of life, and command him — it won't be easy — to leave Angel
alone. "Curb your enthusiasm," he'll say.

Tom's heart will be broken; he'll cling to his mother and cry long
and hard. There won't be any consoling him, no matter how gently
people try to bring his wailing to an end. Everyone will feel awful about
the little tragedy, and people will comfort themselves by saying it's a
"little" tragedy. That's our contempt for children; it's not little for Tom
— it's a real tragedy.

If I'm right about what will happen, I've got self-comforting tricks
to draw on. I'll intellectualize this scene, speculate, philosophize, and
dredge up a story from ancient Greece — except there might not be
one that fits. I'll think fast and come up with something. Now that I
consider it, Thomas Mann's novella *Disorder and Early Sorrow* will fit
the bill. It's the same tale as that of Tom and Angel: a child's poignant
love, inevitable tragedy, and a reminder that childhood love isn't trivial.

Young Tom will have experienced one of the great joys of life and,
like all great joys it will be fleeting. The truly intense joys, thrilling
beyond belief, are: falling in love, having children, passionate involvement in a cause, being dramatically cured. But the final joy must be
more cautious; for me, it's standoffishness, watching. It's the safest
one for me. Intense joys are ephemeral: love fades, children grow up,
causes fail or become corrupt, dramatic cures are temporary or turn
out to be cures by war or hatred. "Oh, dear," is what I say.

Whether it's Thomas Mann's Gustav Aschenbach falling in love
with Tadziu on a Venice beach, Tom falling in love with Angel, or you
or me falling in love and having broken hearts, doesn't matter. Nor
does it matter if we never fall in love, or fall in love with books or birds
or bicycles; we're all placebo competent — wrong words, rather,
placebo inevitable. We can't live without broken hearts, vitamin pills,
and student protests, whichever of the things we do that brings us
alive. We think technology — grief counseling, psychotherapy, pills —
can spare us, but they only work for a moment.

✣ ✣ ✣

A half hour has passed and I'm munching my last baguette. My second espresso will be here momentarily. I'm luxuriating one last time in Provence's sun and warmth and, as usual, there are thirty to forty sunbathers abandoning themselves to their own beauty around the pool, heedless of warnings against the sun, more joyous in their own bodies and clothes than people in Toronto. Most are women, young mothers whose children are in the pool, and nearly all of whom wear tiny bikini swimsuits. Beside me is a pretty woman—she's barely twenty-five, with lovely tanned skin and a hearty pregnant tummy. Her belly button sports a gold ring that sticks out merrily. On the other side is her little daughter, who has a matching, equally fine round tummy.

On the porch, people eat and chatter incomprehensibly — I don't understand a word of French — and others head for the tennis courts. To my left is a beach-volley-ball court, where, as he does every day, a coach trains two athletic-looking young women. They are better play-ers than he, but, morning and evening, he drills them mercilessly, obviously preparing them for some match or tournament. The young women also wear bikinis but the colours of their skimpy swimsuits seem to represent their teams; they wear matching baseball hats, obligatory ponytails poking out at the back.

Many people on the porch are smoking, and my waitress's chubby fingers flaunt numerous gold-coloured rings; her neck and wrists are also bedecked with plenty of gold chains, bracelets, and little medal-lions. These are real people; they cheer me and prove my point: the ceremonies they practise keep their souls in tip-top condition. In con-sequence, when I think about placebos, I no longer have to think they're silly or fake.

Sadly and secretly, you and I know that, when the mood is upon them, these fabulous people are also stupid, cowardly, and evil. That cures them, too — of something. It's stuff people does.

※ ※ ※

Philippe, the manager of Sunset Village, is the only person who speaks English; the staff are as indifferent to my English as I am to their

French. These French people are *French*, of course, and I like it that they're so fixed on being who they are. Like the French, half the world fulfills itself (I'm sneaking in the placebo topic again) by celebrating their uniqueness and individuality; the other half lives in the intoxicating dream that the Self can dissolve in the All. Since the Second World War, Germans, my blood kin, seem to have fit themselves into the latter category.

I worry about my fellow Germans; when I visit Germany they instantly hear my accent and switch to English. I'd fall over if, here in France, I heard people jabbering away in English. I bitch when I'm in Germany because I want to practise my German, and they explain that they are being polite. But I'll bet five cents, five dollars, five billion dollars, that they are abasing themselves. It's hard to get over the guilt of the Second World War even for those born years after it ended sixty years ago; Germans think they stand a little outside humanity. So Germans conform, don't make waves, stay conservative, adapt. I hate to admit this, but the Germans are right; they didn't sacrifice their babies as the ancients instructed us to do, so they ended up sacrificing their own souls.

I'll shock you if I say the torturers in the concentration camps aren't my biggest worry, nor are Hitler himself and the thugs close to him. I'm more worried about the people who designed humane gas chambers and those who, out of empathy, put people out of their misery with a bullet in the brain. The humane and the empathic terrify me, because they are ordinary, decent citizens, who, as instructed, have always made burnt offerings, eaten the body and blood of Christ each week, and done their duty. They are the woman on television on August 27, 2004, who says she will vote for George W. Bush because he is the commander-in-chief. When challenged by the interviewer, she didn't offer arguments about policy. "He's the commander-in-chief," she reiterated. Such people terrify me because they are me, and, I'm sorry to add, they are you. An ass like Hitler would never think about such things, nor would he read this book.

When you and I have conservative instincts, when we're conformists and good citizens, we stand in a dangerous place, teetering on the brink of becoming humane thugs. We're like the psychiatrists who are afraid to notice that, since every psychiatric treatment "works," they ought to start thinking about the placebo effect. People like you and me — and Kay Redfield Jamison — are dangerous because we're apt to thoughtlessly go along with popular ideas. Rarely do crazy, weird, or nutty ways matter except as something interesting to notice. And on judgement day, if some people have been disturbingly mad, even if (I'll get the strap for this!) they have killed themselves, it probably won't matter.

But it *does* matter if we say psychiatric patients have biological abnormalities. Well, if modern psychiatrists think psychiatric patients have diseases, they should immediately trot out the evidence. But it better not be the self-hypnotizing "evidence" such as I've cited from the Middle Ages about how to go about identifying a witch or a devil, the so-called "suggestive evidence" that's taken seriously only by those who've sold their souls.

If psychiatrists practise their placebo cures knowingly, they will do no harm. Then, even if I don't approve of their methods — electroconvulsive therapy, phototherapy, juvenile types of psychotherapy, most drugs — I'll have no legitimate complaint. Mostly it's the damn drugs that bother me, putting something into our mouths, since time immemorial the tactic of doctors and charlatans alike. We must have our herbs, vitamins, minerals, and bottled water, it seems. But benign though they may be, it doesn't mean psychiatrists should join in. Why not? Because our job is different: we ought to think about why, when the human spirit aches, it is as easily fixed by Norton Disk Doctor, a sugar pill, or a reassuring smile as by anything else. Psychiatry has need of rituals.

Having lost faith in healing waters, we're left with one safe placebo: psychotherapy. I doubt people are cured of craziness after doing the talking cure with me, but I hope I've made them think — or think again. I can't, of course, cure them of anything, because they haven't got diseases. And I can't make them wise because that depends on them. If they meet with me, I simply do my best to undermine their usual assumptions. Yes, I'm a saboteur, which is not a nice word. I'm courteous and concerned, too, but that's conventional decency, and the harsher word describes the tactic I use to pressure my patients to think.

It's said jokingly that the viciousness of academic disputes is because the stakes are so small. In contrast to scientific, philosophical, and religious conflict, academic disputes in psychiatry barely exist. I conclude that the rituals surrounding mental well-being are so precious that only strange, disgruntled people like me would question established traditions and practices. Their commonest form is prescribing and proscribing the swallowing of special symbolic things: take these pills; don't eat that food. Dare I link this to speech, the mouth-deed that so powerfully defines us as human? Do we fear speaking the truth because it puts our souls in jeopardy?

Many psychiatrists won't like it if I compare what we do to the treatments devised for another popular epidemic: repetitive strain injuries (RSI). "We're breaking down our bodies," announced an article in this morning's *Globe and Mail*. A sticker on my computer warns me of the same danger: "To reduce the risk of serious injury to hands, wrists, or other joints, read Safety & Comfort Guide." The 2.3 million Canadians who suffer from RSI will be heartened to hear that they can get help from acupressure, sacro-cranial massage, physio, exercises, group encounters, yoga, meditation, acupuncture, an ergonomic desk chair, alternating tasks, stretching, fitness, and warming up before typing. The alternative is to be like me: smug.

When writing, I work on my computer many hours a day, sitting on a kitchen chair; my neck, shoulders, back, arms, and fingers feel fine. I'm still hoping that another self-cure, crabbing about the 2.3 million Canadians who have repetitive strain injuries — and about my psychiatric colleagues — will accomplish something, that I will be freed by wailing about someone else's foibles, curing myself of the woes of life by saying RSI is silly.

Graham Greene tells the story of his family's gardener, a man called Charge. One night Charge got tight and forgot to stoke the stove in the orchid house. All the orchids died, including one for which his father had refused an offer of three hundred pounds, the equivalent today of many thousands of dollars. His father, a school headmaster, must have been devastated, as devastated, says Graham Greene, as *he* would have been if one of his manuscripts were carelessly destroyed. But his father never mentioned the matter, nor was the gardener sacked.

Mr. Greene senior nobly lived out the great British tradition in which he was embedded: the stiff upper lip. No wailing. I'm embedded in a different tradition, a scientific cultural tradition in which I'm not permitted to have a stiff upper lip. In the face of psychiatric folly I'm obliged to wail. Picking on the countless hysterias in which our species indulges, including repetitive strain injury, is a hysteria in its own right. All of us are smug about our own ways and hysterical about the ways of others.

Although it's my professional duty to be critical of psychiatric enthusiasms that need to be curbed, it's also my professional duty to tolerate the cries of anguish of my patients. They all cry out in their own language: depression, RSI, schizophrenia, and alien abduction are symbolic statements of suffering and, simultaneously, indicators of unexpected ways of fitting into our culture; wailing and fitting in are done in many languages. Even my wailing — "people shouldn't wail so much" — is just another piece of humanity in action.

Stanley Walker, once city editor of the New York *Herald Tribune*, puts this in perspective: "existence is primarily a droll affair, with the horse laugh predominant not only to the grave, but after the will is read."[2]

⁛ ⁛ ⁛

There are plenty of good psychiatrists, and in the universities, a small community of fine researchers sticks to basic neuro/molecular/physiological science, valuable to medicine in general but pretty well irrelevant to psychiatry. Such real scientists are harder and harder to see, because their presence is obscured by a primal horde of badly trained researchers, who, in the mistaken belief they are scientists, do useless research. They've taken over university departments of psychiatry. *For heaven's sake*, I say to myself, *it isn't as though we're asking them to conjugate German irregular verbs — just the rudiments of collecting evidence, logic, and theory building.*

Sadly, many good clinicians leave the universities, preferring to work in private offices. They listen to patients, think hard, and worry about their own biases. Yes, the clinicians worry about their own biases. They also exercise their minds: read difficult books, go to movies, play Scrabble, puzzle over moral dilemmas. And, I suspect, without being prodded, they study German irregular verbs: by bulking up intellectually, they become musclemen of the mind. Such doctors watch closely as the radiant oddness of life unfolds.

ACKNOWLEDGEMENTS

I'm grateful for the financial assistance of the Canada Council for the Arts, whose vote of confidence was very welcome; I'm on my own when I write as critically about my profession as I do.

Albert Wong and I have argued for years about biological psychiatry but, despite arguments, hardly disagree. He stirs up my usual habits of thought. Avery Krisman and I talk and think, often agreeing. Together, we shake our heads in amazement at the sorry state of modern psychiatry. My agent and good friend, Denise Bukowski, did double duty as an editor of early drafts of this book. Kevin Linder, Derek Fairbridge, and Pat Kennedy, my editors, pushed me to correct and clarify, patiently nudging me to see inconsistencies in my arguments and awkwardness in my style. I'm grateful to all these committed people.

When my book needs got esoteric, librarians at the CAMH Main Library hunted things down. Sebastian Brandt's *Ship of Fools* prompted Zahra Akhavian and Robyn Mound to widen their eyes, excited by the Albrecht Dürer woodcuts. When I had trouble finding an English-language copy of the *Malleus Maleficarum*, Gary Bell knew where to find it. Most psychiatrists don't know these are basic psychiatric texts.

ENDNOTES

INTRODUCTION

1. Albert Hung Choy Wong and Hubert H. M. Van Tol, "Schizophrenia: From Phenomenology to Neurobiology," *Neuroscience and Biobehavioral Reviews* 27(3) (2003): 269–306.

CHAPTER ONE: THE LOVE AFFAIR WITH SCIENCE

1. Irving Kirsch and David Antonuccio, "Antidepressants Versus Placebos: Meaningful Advantages Are Lacking," *Psychiatric Times,* Vol. xix(9) September, 2002, 6–7.
2. Roger McIntyre et al (11 other authors), "Measuring the Severity of Depression and Remission in Primary Care: Validation of the HAMD-7 Scale," *Canadian Medical Association Journal* 173(11) (November 22, 2005): 1327–34.
3. David Healy, *The Antidepressant Era* (Cambridge: Harvard University Press, 1997).
4. Edward Shorter, *Historical Dictionary of Psychiatry* (Oxford: Oxford University Press, 2005).
5. Robert Whitaker, *Mad in America: Bad Science, Bad Medicine, and the Enduring Mistreatment of the Mentally Ill* (New York: Basic Books, 2002).

CHAPTER TWO: AN EPIDEMIC OF SUPERSTITION

1. Heinrich Institoris, *The Malleus Maleficarum* [of Heinrich Kramer and James Sprenger], trans. Montague Summers (Escondido, CA: The Book Tree, 2000).
2. Nancy C. Andreasen, *Brave New Brain: Conquering Mental Illness in the Era of the Genome* (Oxford: Oxford University Press, 2001).
3. American Psychiatric Association, "Statement on 'Diagnosis and Treatment of Mental Disorders,'" Press release No. 03–39, September 26, 2003.
4. Henri Ellenberger, *The Discovery of the Unconscious: The History and Evolution of Dynamic Psychiatry* (New York: Basic Books, 1970).
5. Jim Windolf, "A Nation of Nuts," *Wall Street Journal*, October 22, 1997.
6. Robert Burton, *The Anatomy of Melancholy* (New York: New York Review of Books, 2001).

7. Charles Rosen, "The Anatomy Lesson," *New York Review of Books*, vol. LII(10) June 9, 2005, 55–59.

8. Arthur Miller, *Timebends* (New York: Grove Press, 1987).

9. American Psychiatric Association, "Statement on 'Diagnosis and Treatment of Mental Disorders,'" Press release No. 03–39, September 26, 2003.

10. David Healy, *The Antidepressant Era* (Cambridge: Harvard University Press, 1997), pp. 98–99.

11. Sigmund Freud, "Mourning and Melancholia," *The Standard Edition of the Complete Psychological Works of Sigmund Freud, Vol. 14* (London: Hogarth Press, 1957).

CHAPTER THREE: DRUGS VERSUS PLACEBOS

1. David Healy, *The Antidepressant Era* (Cambridge: Harvard University Press, 1997).

2. Thomas Mann, *The Magic Mountain*, trans. John E. Woods (New York: Alfred A. Knopf Inc., 1995).

3. Robert Burton, *The Anatomy of Melancholy* (New York: New York Review of Books, 2001).

4. John Cornwell, *The Power to Harm: Mind, Medicine and Murder on Trial* (New York: Viking Press, 1996).

5. Simon Schama, *Rembrandt's Eyes* (New York: Alfred A. Knopf Inc., 1999), pp. 72–73.

6. Marcia Angell, *The Truth About the Drug Companies: How They Deceive Us and What to Do About It* (New York: Random House, 2004).

7. Merrill Goozner, *The $800 Million Pill: The Truth Behind the Cost of New Drugs* (Berkeley: University of California Press, 2005).

8. David Healy, *The Creation of Psychopharmacology* (Cambridge: Harvard University Press, 2004).

9. John Cornwell, *The Power to Harm: Mind, Medicine and Murder on Trial* (New York: Viking Press, 1996).

10. Robert Whitaker, "The Case Against Antipsychotic Drugs: A 50-year Record of Doing More Harm Than Good," *Medical Hypotheses* 62: (2004): 5–13.

11. Robert Whitaker, *Mad in America: Bad Science, Bad Medicine, and the Enduring Mistreatment of the Mentally Ill* (New York: Basic Books, 2002).

12. CBC News, "Woman Awarded $100,000 for CIA-funded Electroshock," June 10, 2004, http://www.cbc.ca/stories/2004/06/10/canada/shock_award040610-(accessed February 2, 2006).

13. René Descartes, "Principles of Philosophy IV," *Philosophical Essays and Correspondence* (Cambridge: Hackett Publishing Co., 2000).

14. Richard Lewontin, *The Triple Helix: Gene, Organism, and Environment* (Cambridge: Harvard University Press, 2002), p. 17.

CHAPTER FOUR: THE FALLACY OF SPECIFIC CAUSES

1. Thomas Szasz, *The Myth of Mental Illness: Foundations of a Theory of Personal Conduct* (New York: Harper and Row, 1984).
2. Kay Redfield Jamison, *Night Falls Fast: Understanding Suicide* (New York: Alfred A. Knopf Inc., 1999).
3. Newscast on Canadian Broadcasting Corporation, April 2, 2000.
4. John Steinbeck, *The Grapes of Wrath* (New York: Viking Press, 1989).
5. Leo Tolstoy, *War and Peace*, 2nd ed., ed. and trans. George Gibian (New York: W. W. Norton & Co., 1996).

CHAPTER SEVEN: FEASTING AND FASTING

1. Peter T. Katzmarzyk, "The Canadian Obesity Epidemic, 1985–1998," *The Canadian Medical Association Journal* 166 (8), (April 16, 2002).

CHAPTER EIGHT: AFFIRMING WHO WE ARE

1. Ernest Jones, *The Life and Work of Sigmund Freud, Vol. III* (New York: Basic Books, 1957), p. 164.
2. Anita Diamant, *The Red Tent* (New York: A Wyatt Book for St. Martin's Press, 1997).

CHAPTER NINE: DECENCY, VIRTUE, RIGHTEOUSNESS

1. Hermann Kurzke, *Thomas Mann: Life as a Work of Art*, trans. Leslie Willson (Princeton: Princeton University Press, 2002), p. 489.

CHAPTER ELEVEN: BEAUTY, TASTE, THE ARTS

1. Richard Smith, "Editorial: Spend (Slightly) Less on Health and More on the Arts," *British Medical Journal.* 325 (December 21, 2002) 1432–1433.
2. Vladimir Vladimirovich Nabokov, *Pale Fire* (New York: Ardis, 1983).
3. Graham Greene, *A Burnt-out Case* (London: Heinemann, 1961), p. 118.

CHAPTER TWELVE: RESHAPING THE SOUL

1. Robert Hughes, *Culture of Complaint: The Fraying of America* (Oxford: Oxford University Press, 1993).
2. Wendy Kaminer, *I'm Dysfunctional, You're Dysfunctional: The Recovery Movement and Other Self-Help Fashions* (New York: Addison-Wesley, 1992).

CHAPTER THIRTEEN: EVERYTHING WORKS

1. Roger McIntyre et al (11 other authors), "Measuring the Severity of Depression and Remission in Primary Care: Validation of the HAMD-7 Scale," *Canadian Medical Association Journal* 173(11) (November 22, 2005).

CHAPTER FOURTEEN: CHANGING THE THEORIES WE LIVE BY

1. American Psychiatric Association, "Statement on 'Diagnosis and Treatment of Mental Disorders,'" Press release No. 03–39, September 26, 2003.
2. Stephen Vizinczey, *Truth and Lies in Literature* (London: Hamish Hamilton Ltd., 1986).
3. Richard Dawkins, *The Blind Watchmaker: Why the Evidence of Evolution Reveals a Universe Without Design* (New York: W. W. Norton & Co., 1985).
4. René Spitz, *Anaclitic Depression* (New York: International Universities Press, 1946).

CHAPTER FIFTEEN: PLACEBO: THE SECRET HEALER

1. Emily Dickinson, *The Complete Poems of Emily Dickinson*, ed. Thomas Johnson, J70 (Toronto: Little, Brown and Co., 1924).

CHAPTER SIXTEEN: RADIANT ODDNESS

1. Thomas Mann, *Doctor Faustus: The Life of the German Composer Adrian Leverkühn, as Told by a Friend*, trans. H. T. Lowe-Porter (New York: Alfred A. Knopf Inc., 1948).
2. Russell Baker, "Review: A Great Reporter at Large," *New York Review of Books* vol. 51 (18) (November 18, 2004).

INDEX

Achilles, 40, 143, 167, 184, 206
acupuncture, 78, 130
Adam and Eve, 116, 144
addiction, 31, 49–50
adultery, 184
aesthetic healing, 204, 205, 206
aestheticism, 202–211
affirmation, 154–70
   gender, 156, 167
   in men, 156, 157, 166–67
   and sexual activity, 159, 163
   in women, 155–56, 157, 169
African masculinity rituals, 166–67
agency, 87, 97–102
aging, 88
Ahab, Captain, 206
alcohol, 153
alcoholism, 31, 49
Ali, Muhammad, 39, 156
Allan Memorial Institute, 69
Almodóvar, Pedro, 125
Alzheimer's disease, 29
American Journal of Psychiatry, 2, 24
American Psychiatric Association,
   25, 39, 249
Americans, 31, 42, 152
Anatomy of Melancholy, The (Burton),
   33–34, 58, 91–92
ancient Greece,
   átā, 98, 189, 194
   beliefs, 52, 97, 148
   mythology, 144–46, 179, 182
   teachers, 147
   theories about madness, 2, 24, 27, 248
Angell, Marcia, 62
animal magnetism, 28
animism, 214
anorexia nervosa, 87, 118, 145–46, 149,
   151–52
Antidepressant Era, The (Healy), 56, 63
antidepressants
   for anxiety, 47

clinical trials, 46
culture and use, 46
effect of, 12–13
excessive number, 62
flawed studies, 63
future of, 69
NSRIS, 62
placebo effect, 12–13, 57, 129, 232
promotion, 56
Prozac, 43, 45, 46, 47, 56, 65–66
side effects, 12–13, 148
SSRIS, 46
Tofranil (imipramine), 56–57, 62, 63
anti-psychiatry movement, 25, 104,
   132, 133
antipsychotic (neuroleptic) drugs,
   47, 67–68, 69, 194, 196
Antony and Cleopatra (Shakespeare),
   77, 79
anxiety, 15, 47, 83, 261
anxiolytics, 46
art, 202–204, 207
artists, 202–203
átā, 98, 189, 194
atropine, 13
attention deficit disorder, 31, 60, 87,
   130, 198
Auden, W. H., 3, 193
Aunt Dona, 168–69, 260–61

Baker, Josephine, 39
Batman, 40, 143
Baumann, Ralph, 123–24, 133, 142
Beck Depression Inventory (BDI), 65, 82
behaviourism, 162
Believers and Skeptics, 189–91
Bernheim, Hippolyte, 28
Bible, 144, 169, 278
biological causes of mental disorder,
   lack of, 2, 4, 17, 24–25, 249
biological psychiatrists, 30, 35, 36,
   60–61, 88–89, 97

biological research, 65
biology metaphor, 79
Bittschwamm Salbe, 129
blaming, 173, 185, 217, 221, 263
Blind Watchmaker, The (Dawkins), 252
blood, 78, 145, 146, 169, 170
bloodletting (bleeding), 38, 58, 78
Blumhardt, Reverend, 156–57
Boots, Rick, 220–21
borderline personality disorder, 31, 104,
    240, 263, 268
Boujoff, George, 242
Bovary, Emma (Madame), 39, 184, 206
boys, feminization of, 167
"brain mythology," 29
brain syphilis (neurosyphilis), 15, 29, 46
Brecht, Bertolt, 263
British culture, 35, 36, 287
British Medical Journal, 207
Broad, Dr., 259, 260, 262
broken heart, 188, 282
Buddha, 208, 209, 224, 242
Burke, Tony, 173–81, 182–83
Burnt-out Case, A (Greene), 210
Burton, Robert, 33, 34, 58, 91, 92

Cameron, Ewan, 69
CAMH. *See* Centre for Addiction and
    Mental Health
Campbell, "Soupy," 123
Canadians, 152, 226, 286
Cape Town (South Africa), 166
Carrey, Jim, 17
case reports,
    Burke, Tony, 173–81, 182–83
    Clement, Jane (Mrs.), 146–49, 150,
        271–75
    Eisen, Donnie, 140–43, 150, 265
    Keyuan, Yang, 41–43, 132, 167
    Sawanas, Debbie, 135–39
    Yes-No, Agnes, 218–19
causality, 18, 59, 72, 93, 94
causal theory, 2, 98, 102
CBT. *See* cognitive behaviour therapy
celibacy, 125
Centre for Addiction and Mental Health
    (CAMH), 24, 104, 161, 174
ceremonies and rituals,
    addiction and, 50

cultural, 38, 86, 166–67, 192
    food, 150, 152
    habits, 140
    human actions as, 45
    Mayan, 151
    medical, 13–14, 57, 83, 192, 244
    and placebo cures, 38, 48,
        70–72, 119, 190
    in psychiatry, 4, 58, 194, 207
    sexual activity and, 159, 163, 166, 169
    traditional view, 48
    treatments, 59, 192, 194, 204, 262
    way of life, 181, 189
Cervantes, Miguel, 234
chaos theory, 108, 258
Chopra, Deepak, 46, 47
Christianity, 117, 214
chronic fatigue syndrome, 17, 31, 40–41,
    42, 60, 191
cleansing,
    colonic irrigation, 13, 123–24, 133, 142
    fasting, 118
    as placebo cure, 70, 129
    steam bath, 127–28
    Turkish haircut, 126–27
Clement, Jane (Mrs.), 146–49, 150,
    271–75
Cleopatra, 77, 79, 82, 277–78
clinical trials, 46
Cody, John, 261
cognitive behaviour therapy (CBT), 47,
    65, 162, 240, 258
Collins, John Churton, 18
colonic irrigation, 13, 123–24, 133, 142
co-morbidity, 114–16
Conrad, Joseph, 265
Cook, Sally, 135, 136, 137, 218
Cordelia, 179, 246, 251, 253, 257
Cornwell, John, 66
"crazy," 51, 193, 265
Crucible, The (Miller), 37
cultists, 226
culture,
    antidepressants and, 46
    depression and, 42, 46
    placebo effect and, 42, 45
    psychiatry and, 98, 215, 216, 218, 268
    psychoanalysis and, 194
    symptoms of, 42

Culture of Complaint (Hughes), 216
Cunning Little Vixen, The (Janáček),
        204–205, 206–207
cures. *See* placebos *and* treatment
cystic fibrosis, 103

Dawkins, Richard, 252
dementia praecox, 29. *See also*
        schizophrenia
Demeter, 144
demon possession, 2, 109, 156, 214–15,
        221
depression. *See also* antidepressants
    adolescents and, 160–61
    Beck Depression Inventory, 65, 82
    "causes," 30
    claimed neurochemistry of, 25
    culture and, 42, 46
    "disease," 4, 57, 82, 103
    electroshock therapy for, 44
    genes, 4, 86
    Hamilton Rating Scale, 63, 65, 82
    history, 58
    inability to measure, 13
    Jamison's theories on, 85, 86, 103
    lifestyle, 87, 94
    prevalency of, 17, 31, 47, 51, 56
    questionnaires for, 82
    synonyms, 15
    treatment of, 13, 56, 57, 240
Descartes, 72
Diagnostic and Statistical Manual. See
        DSM-IV
Diamant, Anita, 169
Dickinson, Emily, 268
Dietrich, Marlene, 39
Discovery of the Unconscious, The
        (Ellenberger), 28
disease,
    categories, 60
    depression as, 4, 57, 82, 103
    euphemism, 30
    idea of, 76
    Koch's Postulates and, 80
    mental disorders as, 4, 79, 243
    metaphors, 36, 268
    psychiatry and, 46, 76, 79, 81, 83
    schizophrenia as, 2, 4, 60
    social construct, 88

    suicide and, 104
Disorder and Early Sorrow (Mann), 282
disorders. *See also names of individual*
        disorders
    American statistics, 31
    as "diseases," 4, 79, 243
    dissociative, 32
    functional, 86–87
    lack of evidence for biological cause,
        2, 4, 17, 24–25, 249
    media, 31–32
    reactions to, 193–94
    trends in, 17
Dittus, Gottliebin, 156–57
divine infatuation (*átā*), 98, 189, 194
doctors,
    faith in, 6, 13
    as healers, 279
    science and, 22
Dona (Aunt), 168–69, 260–61
Don Quixote, 116–17
doublethink, 52–53, 101
drug companies, 58, 59, 62–63, 65–67
drugs. *See also* antidepressants
    addiction, 49, 50
    antipsychotic (neuroleptic), 47, 67–68,
        69, 194, 196
    atropine, 13
    behaviour changes from, 68
    disease categories and, 60
    imipramine (Tofranil), 56–57, 62, 63
    lithium, 68
    NSRIS, 62
    placebo effect, 68
    Prozac (fluoxetine), 43, 45, 46, 47, 56,
        65–66
    science and, 59
    side effects, 12–13, 47, 66, 67, 257
    SSRIS, 46
    symptoms, 73–74
    tranquilizers, 46
    Valium, 46, 47, 81
    vs. placebos, 54–75
DSM-IV, 39, 79
dynamic psychotherapy. *See* psycho-
        analysis

Eastwood, Clint, 40, 125
eating customs, 150–52

Echo, 179
Eisen, Donnie, 140–43, 150, 265
electroshock treatment, 44–45, 46, 132,
    133, 257
Eli Lilly and Company, 59, 65–66
Ellenberger, Henri, 28
empiricism, 18, 19, 47, 197
euphemisms, 30, 89, 195, 196, 243, 276
evidence, 11, 54
expectation, 27
experts, 6
extrasensory perception, 90–91

fasting, 71, 118, 205
Faust, 277, 281
Ferenczi, Sandor, 163–65
fibromyalgia, 41, 57, 83, 130, 191, 198
Fine, Les, 127
fluoxetine. See Prozac
food,
    eating customs, 150–52
    Eisen, Donnie, and, 140–43
    fasting, 71, 118, 205
    gagging on, 148
    in Greek mythology, 144–46
    sacrifice and, 152
    tradition and, 152–53
foramen, 93, 94
four humours, 77–78, 80
Frayn, Doug, 242
free-association, 38, 113
free will, 89, 94, 102
Freud, Sigmund,
    Ferenczi, Sandor, and, 164
    methods, 191
    pathogenic secrets, 199
    as a "poet," 25
    prescription for hysteria, 163
    psychiatric views, 29, 30, 120
    publications by, 48, 119
functional disorders, 86–87

gagging, 148
Garma, Angel, 97
Gates, Bill, 206
gender roles, 155–57, 159, 167, 184
genes,
    creativity and, 5

cystic fibrosis and, 103
depression and, 4, 30
evolution and, 252
homosexuality and, 253
psychiatric disorders and, 60, 103
schizophrenia and, 90, 253
suicide and, 86
Germany, 222, 261, 284
Godfather, The, 40
Goethe, 55, 221
Goozner, Merrill, 63
Grapes of Wrath, The (Steinbeck), 87
Greece, ancient. See ancient Greece
Greene, Graham, 210, 286–87
group anxiety, 261
guilt, defeating, 109–121
    dietary practices and, 117–18
    eating and, 144
    placebos for, 120
    purification, 118
    self-mutilation, 119

habits, 49, 50
Hades, 144, 145, 182
Haiti, 256
Hamilton, Max, 63
Hamilton Rating Scale for Depression,
    63, 64, 82
Hamlet, 51, 116, 201
happiness, 68
healers, 136, 137
Healy, Dr. David, 46, 56, 63, 64–65
heart, broken, 188, 282
Heart of Darkness (Conrad), 265
Helen of Troy, 39, 184
Herodotus, 55
Hippocrates, 24
Historical Dictionary of Psychiatry
    (Shorter), 14
homosexuality, 48, 143, 167, 184, 253, 278
Hughes, Robert, 216
Hulk, 206
humours of the body, 77–78, 80
hydrotherapy, 195
hypnosis, 231–32
hypotheses, 247–48, 250–51, 254
hysteria, 38–40

Illarionovich Kozlov, Nikolai, 93, 94
imbalance, 82
I'm Dysfunctional, You're Dysfunctional
    (Kaminer), 216
imipramine (Tofranil), 56–57, 62, 63
impotence, 158, 185, 186
in-depth psychotherapy. *See* psycho-
    analysis
indeterminism, 102
India, 227
Inge, George, 109–110
In Praise of Older Women (Vizinczey), 250
insulin-coma treatment, 44, 69, 224
"Integrative Psychotherapy," 232–33
interpersonal therapy (IPT), 47, 162, 258
Isherwood, Christopher, 202

Jamison, Dr. Kay Redfield, 85–89,
    91–92, 99, 101–104
Janáček, Leoš, 204, 205
Japan, 46
Jenufa (Janáček), 205
Joan of Arc, 5
Johnson, Samuel, 19
Jung, Carl, 46, 47

Kaminer, Wendy, 216
Keyuan, Yang, 41–43, 132, 167
King Lear (Shakespeare), 116, 224, 251
Koch, Robert, 64, 80
Koch's Postulates, 80, 82, 104, 197
Koran, 169
Kraepelin, Emil, 29, 30
Kramer, Henry, 21
Kraus, Karl, 80
"Kreutzer Sonata, The" (Tolstoy),
    171–72, 173
Kurzke, Hermann, 185

Lansdowne House, 134–35, 139, 218–20,
    255–56
Laws, The (Plato), 243
Lear, King, 179, 225, 246, 251
Lewin, Peter, 219
Lewontin, Richard, 72
Lieberman, Dr. Jeffrey A., 2
lithium, 68
Little Red Riding Hood, 224, 274

Mad in America (Whitaker), 18
madness. *See* schizophrenia
Magic Mountain, The (Mann), 58
Maharaji, 227–230, 233–34
male hysterics, 39–40
Malleus Maleficarum, The (Kramer and
    Sprenger), 22, 185
manic-depressive illness, 29, 31
Mann, Thomas, 58, 77, 185, 234, 281, 282
Marconi, Mike, 174
"master narratives," 255
materialism, 197
materialistic psychiatry, 30
Maximen and Reflexionen (Goethe), 55
Mayans, 214, 216, 217, 218
Mays, John Bentley, 89
McCarthy Senate hearings, 37
McGillivray, Bill, 97
Me, Myself, and Irene, 17–18
media disorders, 31–32
medical ceremonies, 13–14, 57, 83, 192,
    244
Medical Hypotheses, 67
medicine men, 136, 137
Medusa, 125, 129, 182
melancholy, 33–34. *See also* depression
men,
    adultery and, 184
    gender roles, 157–58, 159, 167
    hysteria and, 39–40
    impotence, 158, 185, 186
    sexual fears, 42, 183
Menninger Clinic, 109
Menninger, Karl, 241
menstruation, 125, 169
mental disorders. *See also names of*
        individual disorders
    American statistics, 31
    as "diseases," 4, 79, 243
    lack of evidence for biological cause,
        2, 4, 17, 24–25, 249
    reactions to, 193–94
    trends in, 17
Mesmer, Anton, 28
Metamorphoses (Ovid), 206
metaphor,
    concretizing, 15, 30, 36, 72
    description of, 79

disease and, 36, 268
"imbalance" as 82
psychoanalysis and, 80
mêtis, 194
Miller, Arthur, 37
mimesis, 47, 48
mind–body dualism, 93
Moby Dick (Melville), 206
Monroe, Marilyn, 39
morality, 171–86
Mourning and Melancholia (Freud), 48
multiple chemical sensitivities, 31, 41, 60
multiple personality disorder, 17, 32, 39,
    41, 191, 268
Mustard, Bill, 52
Myth of Mental Illness, The (Szasz), 79
mythology, 29, 143–46, 179, 182

Nabokov, Vladimir, 93, 209
Narcissus, 179
National Academy of Sciences, 31
National Alliance for the Mentally Ill,
    17–18
National Institutes of Health, 63
nature/nurture question, 92
neurasthenia, 40, 42, 86, 132. See also
    chronic fatigue syndrome
neuroleptic (antipsychotic) drugs, 47,
    67–68, 69, 194, 196
Neuroscience and Biobehavioral Reviews, 2
neurosyphilis, 15, 29, 46
neurotransmitters, 24, 25
Nietzsche, 87, 152, 190, 200, 233
Night Falls Fast (Jamison), 85, 103–104, 105
nihilism, 276
nocebos, 26
non-compliance, 104
nonselective monoamine re-uptake
    inhibitors (NSRIS), 62
Nunavut, 86

obsessive-compulsive disorder, 31
Occam's Razor, 115
oddness, 265, 270–88
Odysseus, 145, 157, 173, 184, 224, 264
Odyssey, The (Homer), 98, 144, 264
Oedipus complex, 20, 96, 211, 255

Olympus, 144
orgasms, 147, 148, 159, 186, 229
Ovid, 188, 206

Pale Fire (Nabokov), 209
Parker, Peter, 206
parsimony, 115, 116
pathogenic secrets, 199
penis, 42, 159, 163, 183–84
Persaud, Nadira, 224–25
Persephone, 125, 144–46, 169, 224
personal agency, 87, 97–102
pharmaceutical companies. See drug
    companies
phenomenology, 30
philosophies, 75
phobias, 4, 31, 72, 95, 117, 239, 268
placebo effect,
    antidepressants and, 12–13, 56, 66,
        92, 194
    ceremony and, 38, 48, 192, 230
    cultural differences, 42
    definition, 16
    depression and, 56
    of drugs, 58, 68
    electroshock treatments, 44
    expectation and, 27
    human behaviour and, 16
    on physical ailments, 26, 49, 130, 131,
        192
    in psychiatric treatment, 36, 240, 241
    "real" effect, 19
    research studies and, 16, 59
    suggestion and, 28, 246
    symbolic messages, 138, 139
    on warts, 26, 130
placebos,
    aestheticism, 205
    affirming gender, 159
    antidepressants, 12–13, 46
    of author, 172, 187, 189
    characteristics of, 71
    cleansing, 129
    for chronic fatigue syndrome, 41
    definition, 16, 55
    drugs versus, 54–75
    exorcism, 218

folk remedies, 131
   guilt and, 120
   in history, 58, 78
   lists of, 70–71, 72, 74–75
   for media disorders, 32
   nocebos, 26
   personally designed, 50, 87, 263
   power of, 54
   psychotherapy, 41, 241, 285
   safe, 131, 132, 133, 285
   study of, 59
   and superstition, 55
   as treatment in psychiatry, 7, 16
   versatility of, 205
Plato, 83, 243
Pope Innocent VIII, 21, 22
porphyria, 15
post-traumatic stress disorder, 35, 36,
      83, 85, 217
Potiphar's wife, 169
Power to Harm, The (Cornwell), 66
Pózdnyshev, 171–72, 173
pre-frontal lobotomies, 44
premenstrual dysphoric disorder, 65
Prozac (fluoxetine), 43, 45, 46, 47, 56,
      65–66
psychiatric biology, 46, 47
psychiatric diseases. See mental disorders
      and names of individual disorders
psychiatric drugs. See anti-
      depressants and drugs
psychiatrists,
   biologically oriented, 1, 12, 14, 30, 35, 61
   enchantment, 12
   modern, 27, 29, 30, 34, 87, 105
   ritual and, 80, 84, 105, 212, 271, 273
   role of, 198, 212, 233, 246
   superstitions, 19, 35, 91
psychiatry,
   aesthetics and, 203
   attack on, 79
   ceremony and, 4
   Chinese, 132
   culture and, 98, 215, 216, 218, 268
   defined, 14
   "disease" and, 46, 76, 79, 81, 83
   dynamic, 30, 277

history, 28, 29, 139, 195, 198
   law and, 266, 268
   "master narratives," 255
   materialistic, 30
   metaphors in, 15, 30, 36
   modern, 58
   placebos in, 7, 47, 59, 240–42, 285
   roots of, 24, 25, 27, 199
   "sciences" of, 15
   tests, 64, 81, 242
   theories, 249–50, 252
   treatments, 7, 12, 35, 38, 44, 131–32
   Western, 57, 215
psychoanalysis (dynamic psycho-
      therapy),
   for anxiety, 47
   ceremony and ritual, 194, 225, 271
   as confession, 133
   culture and, 194
   for chronic fatigue syndrome, 41
   defined, 258
   metaphor and, 80
   practice of, 38
   Prozac and, 45
   psychiatry and, 199
   traditional, 226, 240
   as treatment, 239
psychopharmacology, 46, 241
psychotherapy. See also psychoanalysis
   for "borderline" cases, 240
   defined, 41
   dynamic. See psychoanalysis
   learning/teaching, 270, 276
   placebo effect of, 275, 285
   types of, 232, 258
purification, 118, 129

questionnaires, 19, 64, 81, 82

rape, 184
rebirth, 69, 71, 206, 224, 230
Red Tent, The (Diamant), 169
Reil, Johann Christian, 14
religion, 56, 138, 193, 214, 248
repetitive strain injuries (RSIs), 286, 287
rituals. See ceremonies and rituals
Robinson, John, 231, 232

Rosen, Charles, 34
Rutherford, Lord, 79

sacrifice, 144–46, 150–52, 284
Sadiq, Dr. Fahima, 174, 176, 180
Sakel, Manfred, 69
Salomé, 39
Sawanas, Debbie, 135–39
Sawyer, Tom, 26
scales (psychological), 19
Schama, Simon, 61
schizophrenia,
    causal theories, 2, 24
    as "disease," 60
    genetics and, 90, 253
    incidence of, 17
    lack of evidence as brain disease, 2, 4
    as lifestyle, 87
    spectrum disorder, 114
    "suggestive evidence" for, 11
    synonyms for, 15
    treatments for, 44, 47, 69
science, 11–20
    "bad," 12
    definition, 19
    evidence and, 11
    fervour for, 11–12, 59
    medical ceremonies and, 13–14
    placebo effect and, 12–14, 16
    prestige of, 22–23
    superstition and, 36
scientific materialism, 27
scientific method, 246
seasonal affective disorder, 31
selective serotonin re-uptake inhibitors
        (SSRIS), 46
self, affirmation of, 154–70
self-mutilation, 119
Sergeant, Sammy, 129
Seth, Vikram, 158
sex,
    addiction, 31
    intercourse, 136, 159, 163, 179
    metaphor and, 93
    morality and, 182
    mystery of, 144
    orgasms, 147, 148, 159, 186, 229
    patient and psychiatrist, 156

    unprotected, 121
sexist jokes, 163
sexual dysfunction, 186
sexuality, 137, 139
Shakespeare, William, 51, 76, 92, 216,
        264
shamans, 214, 215, 217, 221
Shorter, Edward, 14
Shugar, Gerry, 279
"sick" metaphor, 36
side effects, 12–13, 47, 66, 67, 257
skeptics, 23, 32, 189–91, 248
skull trepanning, 57
smoking, 49, 119
Socrates, 203
Sopranos, The, 40, 116, 200
soul, 212–35
Speak, Memory (Nabokov), 93
spectrum disorders, 114–15
Spiderman, 40, 206
Sprenger, James, 21
SSRIS, 46
Steinbeck, John, 87
Stipec, Joe, 130, 131
stone of folly, 57
style of life, 87, 94
sugar pills. See placebos
"suggestion" hypothesis, 28–29
"suggestive evidence," 5, 11, 89, 285
suicide, 85, 86, 99, 104, 201,
        242–43
Suitable Boy, A (Seth), 158
Summers, Montague, 22
superstition,
    blind belief in science as, 36
    definitions, 20, 36, 48
    epidemic of, 21–53
    guilt and, 144
    in psychiatry, 91, 92
surgery, 26
symptoms, 73–74
    and culture, 42
    depressive, 4, 160
    medical, 16
    painful, 72, 256
    pool of, 42
    psychiatric, 56, 73–74, 115
    withdrawal, 67

synonyms, 15
Szasz, Thomas, 79, 266

Talk to Her, 125
theories,
    ancient Greek, 2, 24, 27, 248
    causal, 2, 98, 102
    changing, 246–58
    nature of, 103
    personal agency, 87, 97–102
    scientific method and, 246–47
    value of, 101
Thomas Mann: Life as a Work of Art
        (Kurzke), 185–86
Tofranil (imipramine), 56–57, 62, 63
Tolstoy, Leo, 90, 171
Toronto General Hospital, 130
tranquilizers, 46
transformation, 203, 206, 231
trauma, 35
travelling, 222, 223
treatment. See also placebos
    author's methods, 84
    ceremonial/ritual, 48, 59, 192, 194,
        204, 262
    for depression, 56, 57, 240
    electroshock, 44–45, 46, 132, 133, 257
    insulin-coma, 44, 69, 224
    psychiatric, 7, 12, 35, 38, 44, 131–32
    psychoanalysis, 239
    for schizophrenia, 44, 47, 69
    travelling as, 223
trepanning, 57
trichotillomania, 110–14, 115, 117

Trilling, Lionel, 97
Triple Helix, The (Lewontin), 72–73
Trudeau, Pierre, 39
Truth About the Drug Companies, The
        (Angell), 62
Twain, Mark, 242

vagina, 118, 125, 168, 169, 182–84
Valium, 46, 47, 81
Van Tol, Hubert, 2
Viagra, 158, 159, 185
virtue, 174, 178
Vizinczey, Stephen, 250
voodoo, 26, 248, 214, 233

Walker, Stanley, 287
War and Peace (Tolstoy), 90
warts, 26, 130
Welsh, Peter, 259, 260
Wesbecker, Joseph, 66
Whitaker, Robert, 18, 67
Wilde, Oscar, 46, 224
Windolf, Jim, 31
witches, 21, 22
Wittgenstein, 71, 87, 88, 94, 95, 96
women
    affirmation in, 155–56, 157, 169
    hysteria and, 38–40
Wong, Albert, 2

Yes-No, Agnes, 218–19

Zeus, 98, 125, 143, 179, 184

Permission is gratefully acknowledged to reprint excerpts from the following:

(pp. 63, 65) Reprinted by permission of the publishers from *The Antidepressant Era* by David Healy, pp. 98–99, Cambridge, Mass.: Harvard University Press, Copyright © 1997 by the President and Fellows of Harvard College.

(p. 73) Reprinted by permission of the publisher from *The Triple Helix* by Richard Lewontin, p. 17, Cambridge, Mass.: Harvard University Press, Copyright © 1998 by Gius, Laterza & Figli Spa, Copyright © 2000 by the President and Fellows of Harvard College.

(p. 164) *The Life and Work of Sigmund Freud, Vol. III* by Ernest Jones (Basic Books, 1957). Used by courtesy of Perseus Books Group.

(pp. 207–208) "Editorial: Spend (Slightly) Less on Health and More on the Arts" by Richard Smith, in *British Medical Journal* 325 (December 21, 2002), pp. 1432–1433. Reproduced with permission from the BMJ Publishing Group.

(pp. 210–211) *A Burnt-out Case* by Graham Greene (Heinemann, 1961). Used by permission of David Higham Associates.

(p. 263) "Mack the Knife." English words by Marc Blitzstein. Original German words by Bert Brecht. Music by Kurt Weill. © 1928 Universal Edition © 1955 Weill-Brecht-Harms Co., Inc. Renewal rights assigned to the Kurt Weill Foundation for Music, Bert Brecht and Edward and Josephine Davis, as Executors of the Estate of Marc Blitzstein. All rights reserved. Used by permission.

(p. 268) Reprinted by permission of the publishers and the Trustees of Amherst College from *The Poems of Emily Dickinson*, Thomas H. Johnson, ed., J70, Cambridge, Mass.: The Belknap Press of Harvard University Press, Copyright © 1951, 1955, 1979, 1983 by the President and Fellows of Harvard College.

Every reasonable effort has been made to contact the holders of copyright for materials quoted in this work. The publishers will gladly receive information that will enable them to rectify any inadvertent errors or omissions in subsequent editions.